Consultants

Carla Gleaton, PT, MEd
PTA Program Director
Kilgore Community College
Kilgore, Texas

David B. Jenkins, PhD
Associate Professor and Head
Section of Anatomy
Southern Illinois University
Alton, Illinois

Robert C. Manske PT, DPT, SCS, MEd, ATC, CSCS
Associate Professor
Department of Physical Therapy
Wichita State University
Wichita, Kansas

Aaron Nevdal PT, DPT
Therapist
Northern Rehab Orthopedic Sports
    Physical Therapy
DeKalb, Illinois

Roberta Kuchler O'Shea, PT, PhD
Associate Professor
Physical Therapy
Governors State University
University Park, Illinois

Kenneth A. Olson, PT, DHSc, OCS, FAAOMPT
Adjunct Faculty, Department of
    Physical Therapy
Northern Illinois University
Therapist
Northern Rehab Orthopedic Sports
    Physical Therapy
DeKalb, Illinois

Derrick Sueki, DPT, GCPT, OCS, AAOMPT
Adjunct Orthopedic Faculty
Mount Saint Mary's College
Adjunct Clinical Faculty, Instructor,
    Clinical Mentor, Orthopedic
    Residency Program
University of Southern California,
    Department of Physical Therapy
Co-President and Director of Physical
    Therapy
Clinical Director and Coordinator of
    Clinical Education
Knight Physical Therapy Inc.
Los Angeles, California

Wolfgang Vogel, MS, PhD
Professor Emeritus
Department of Pharmacology
Jefferson Medical College
Thomas Jefferson University
Philadelphia, Pennsylvania
Adjunct Professor
Florida Gulf Coast University
Fort Meyers, Florida

MOSBY'S

This book is due for return on or before the last date shown below.

MOSBY
ELSEVIER

11830 Westline Industrial Drive
St. Louis, Missouri 63146

Mosby's Field Guide to Physical Therapy   ISBN: 978-0-323-06386-9

Notice

Knowledge and best practice in physical therapy are constantly changing. As new research and experience broaden our knowledge, changes in practice, treatment, and drug therapy may become necessary or appropriate. Readers are advised to check the most current information provided (i) on procedures featured or (ii) by the manufacturer of each product to be administered, to verify the recommended dose or formula, the method and duration of administration, and contraindications. It is the responsibility of the practitioner, relying on their own experience and knowledge of the patient, to make diagnoses, to determine dosages and the best treatment for each individual patient, and to take all appropriate safety precautions. To the fullest extent of the law, the Publisher does not assume any liability for any injury and/or damage to persons or property arising out of or related to any use of the material contained in this book.

ISBN: 978-0-323-06386-9

Vice President and Publisher: Linda Duncan
Executive Editor: Kathy Falk
Senior Developmental Editor: Christie M. Hart
Publishing Services Manager: Julie Eddy
Senior Project Manager: Andrea Campbell
Design Direction: Charlie Seibel

Last digit is the print number: 9   8   7   6   5   4   3   2   1

Printed in Canada

Introduction

As a busy therapist or student in the clinic, having information at your fingertips is important. This field guide gives you quick reference to information commonly needed in practice—providing information on anatomy, assessment tools, screening tools, and much more in a quick-reference format to use for assessment and application, documentation, client education, or communication with clients and other health care professionals.

Mosby's Field Guide to Physical Therapy is a unique handheld reference designed to assist the PT student and clinician, regardless of level of experience, with the basics of point-of-care assessment and treatment. On a daily basis, therapists need information on anatomy and physiology, precautions, applications, assessment pathology and pain, as well as record-keeping. Rather than flip through numerous large texts between clients, this book consolidates key information into one convenient, well-organized, portable guide for fast and easy lookup. The material in this field guide is compiled from leading textbooks and resources for physical therapy and other health care disciplines. Designed as a practical quick reference to assist the physical therapist in practice, it covers the preferred practice pattern key areas: musculoskeletal, neuromuscular, cardiovascular and pulmonary, and integumentary.

Mosby's Field Guide to Physical Therapy will serve as the much-needed resource for students to guide them during clinical course work, for new therapists entering practice, and to physical therapy assistant (PTA) programs because students in these programs must also be able to demonstrate competencies related to their basic practice skills.

Contents

Anatomy

Bones

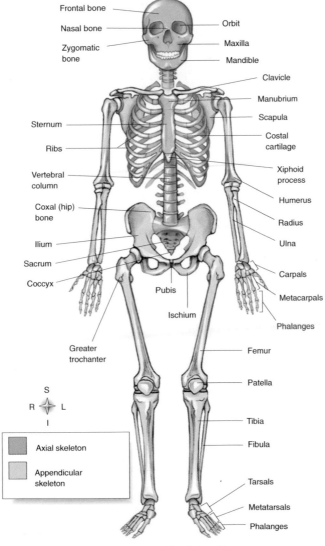

Frontal bone
Nasal bone
Zygomatic bone
Orbit
Maxilla
Mandible
Clavicle
Manubrium
Scapula
Sternum
Costal cartilage
Ribs
Xiphoid process
Vertebral column
Humerus
Coxal (hip) bone
Radius
Ilium
Ulna
Sacrum
Coccyx
Carpals
Pubis
Metacarpals
Ischium
Phalanges
Greater trochanter
Femur
Patella
Tibia
Fibula
Tarsals
Metatarsals
Phalanges

S
R ✛ L
I

Axial skeleton

Appendicular skeleton

Anterior view of the skeleton.[65]

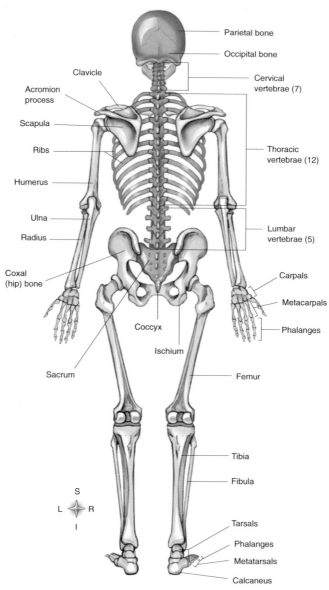

Parietal bone

Occipital bone

Clavicle

Cervical vertebrae (7)

Acromion process

Scapula

Ribs

Thoracic vertebrae (12)

Humerus

Ulna

Radius

Lumbar vertebrae (5)

Coxal (hip) bone

Carpals

Metacarpals

Phalanges

Coccyx

Ischium

Sacrum

Femur

S

L   R

I

Tibia

Fibula

Tarsals

Phalanges

Metatarsals

Calcaneus

Posterior view of the skeleton.[65]

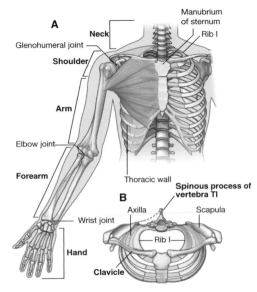

The upper limb. Anterior view of the upper limb (**A**) and superior view of the shoulder (**B**).[19]

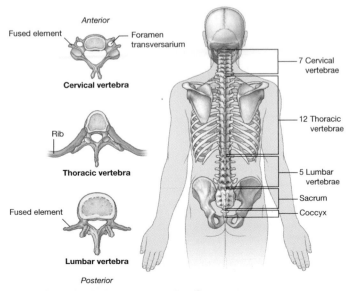

Vertebrae.[19]

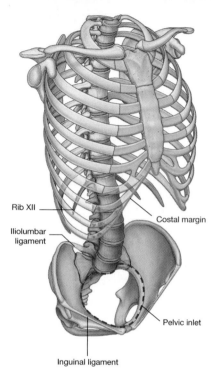

Skeletal elements of the abdominal wall.[19]

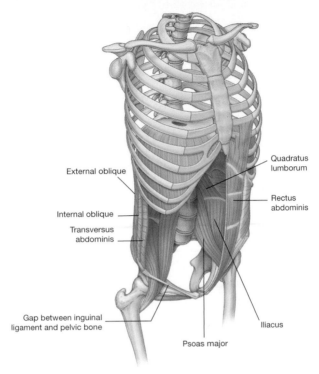

External oblique

Internal oblique

Transversus abdominis

Gap between inguinal ligament and pelvic bone

Quadratus lumborum

Rectus abdominis

Iliacus

Psoas major

Musculoskeletal elements of the abdominal wall.[19]

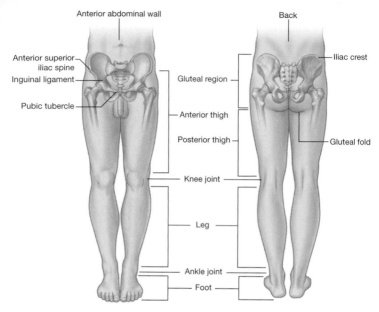

Regions of the lower limb.[19]

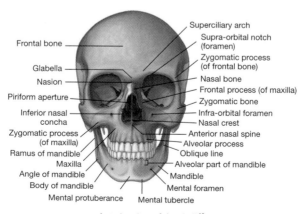

Anterior view of the skull.[19]

Muscles

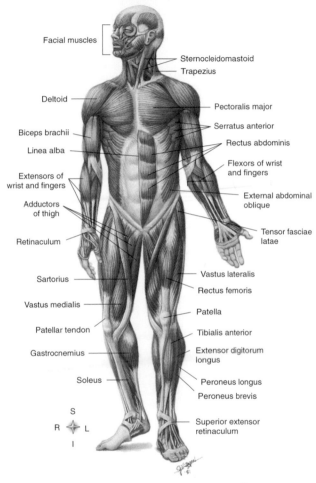

Facial muscles

Sternocleidomastoid

Trapezius

Deltoid

Pectoralis major

Serratus anterior

Biceps brachii

Rectus abdominis

Linea alba

Flexors of wrist and fingers

Extensors of wrist and fingers

External abdominal oblique

Adductors of thigh

Tensor fasciae latae

Retinaculum

Sartorius

Vastus lateralis

Vastus medialis

Rectus femoris

Patella

Patellar tendon

Tibialis anterior

Gastrocnemius

Extensor digitorum longus

Soleus

Peroneus longus

Peroneus brevis

S
R ✦ L
I

Superior extensor retinaculum

Anterior view of the muscles of the body.[65]

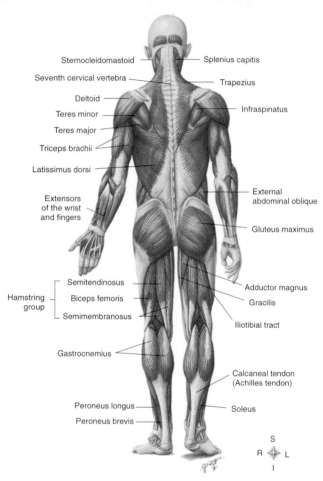

Posterior view of the muscles o the body.[65]

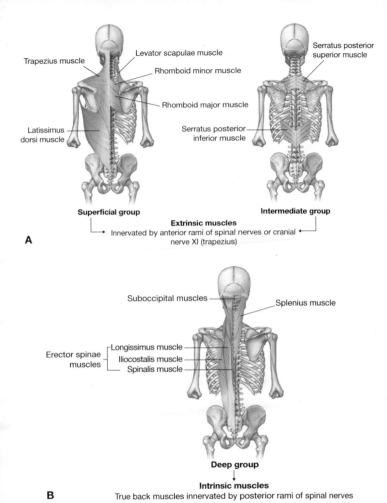

Extrinsic muscles
Innervated by anterior rami of spinal nerves or cranial nerve XI (trapezius)

Intrinsic muscles
True back muscles innervated by posterior rami of spinal nerves

The back muscles. Extrinsic (**A**) and intrinsic (**B**).[19]

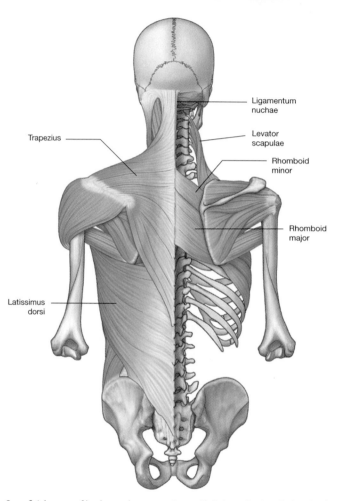

Superficial group of back muscles—trapezius and latissimus dorsi, with rhomboid major, rhomboid minor, and levator scapulae located deep to trapezius in the superior part of the back.[19]

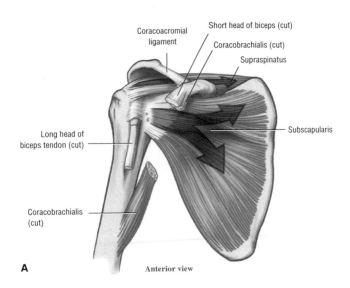

Coracoacromial ligament
Short head of biceps (cut)
Coracobrachialis (cut)
Supraspinatus
Subscapularis
Long head of biceps tendon (cut)
Coracobrachialis (cut)

A   **Anterior view**

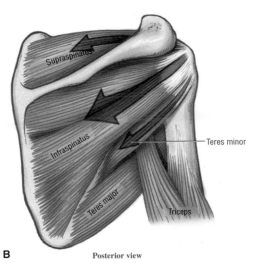

Supraspinatus
Infraspinatus
Teres minor
Teres major
Triceps

B   **Posterior view**

(**A**) Anterior view of the right shoulder, showing the subscapularis muscle blending into the anterior capsule before attaching to the lesser tubercle of the humerus. (**B**) Posterior view of the right shoulder showing the supraspinatus, infraspinatus, and teres minor muscles.[48]

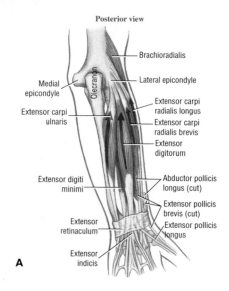

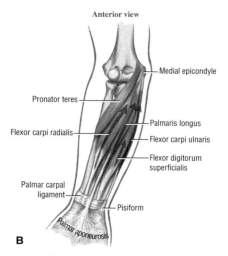

(**A**) Posterior view of the right forearm, showing the primary wrist extensor muscles. (**B**) Anterior view of the right forearm, showing the primary wrist flexor muscles.[48]

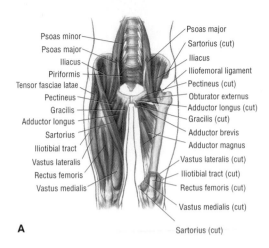

Psoas minor
Psoas major
Iliacus
Piriformis
Tensor fasciae latae
Pectineus
Gracilis
Adductor longus
Sartorius
Iliotibial tract
Vastus lateralis
Rectus femoris
Vastus medialis

Psoas major
Sartorius (cut)
Iliacus
Iliofemoral ligament
Pectineus (cut)
Obturator externus
Adductor longus (cut)
Gracilis (cut)
Adductor brevis
Adductor magnus
Vastus lateralis (cut)
Iliotibial tract (cut)
Rectus femoris (cut)
Vastus medialis (cut)

A

Sartorius (cut)

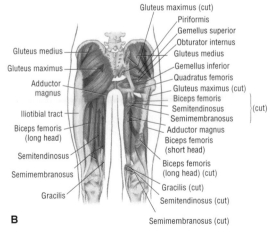

Gluteus medius
Gluteus maximus
Adductor magnus
Iliotibial tract
Biceps femoris (long head)
Semitendinosus
Semimembranosus
Gracilis

Gluteus maximus (cut)
Piriformis
Gemellus superior
Obturator internus
Gluteus medius
Gemellus inferior
Quadratus femoris
Gluteus maximus (cut)
Biceps femoris
Semitendinosus } (cut)
Semimembranosus
Adductor magnus
Biceps femoris (short head)
Biceps femoris (long head) (cut)
Gracilis (cut)
Semitendinosus (cut)
Semimembranosus (cut)

B

(**A**) The anterior muscles of the hip. (**B**) The posterior muscles of the hip.[48]

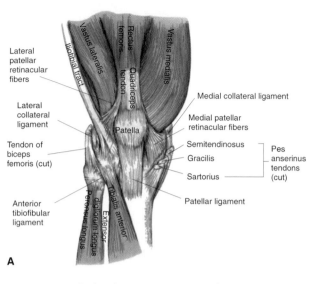

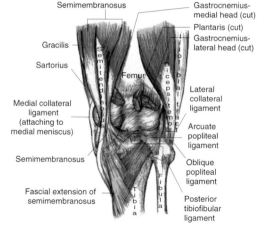

(**A**) Anterior view of the right knee, highlighting many muscles and connective tissues. (**B**) Posterior view of the right knee that emphasizes the major parts of the posterior capsule.[48]

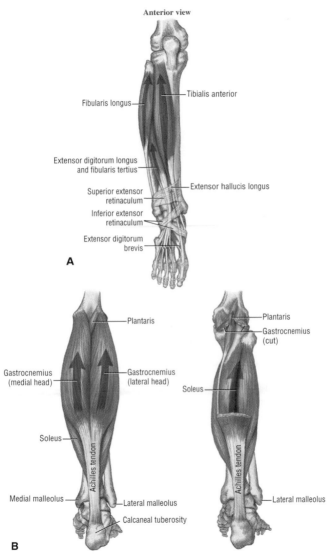

Anterior view

Fibularis longus

Tibialis anterior

Extensor digitorum longus and fibularis tertius

Extensor hallucis longus

Superior extensor retinaculum

Inferior extensor retinaculum

Extensor digitorum brevis

A

Plantaris

Gastrocnemius (medial head)

Gastrocnemius (lateral head)

Soleus

Plantaris

Gastrocnemius (cut)

Soleus

Soleus

Achilles tendon

Medial malleolus

Lateral malleolus

Calcaneal tuberosity

Achilles tendon

Lateral malleolus

B

(**A**) The pretibial muscles of the leg. (**B**) The superficial muscles of the posterior compartment of the right leg.[48]

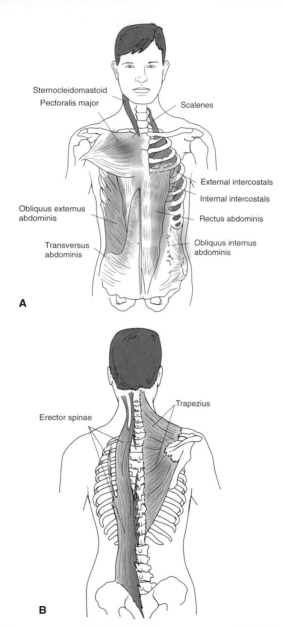

A

B

The respiratory muscles. Anterior view (**A**) and posterior view (**B**).[21]

Organs and Other Anatomical Features

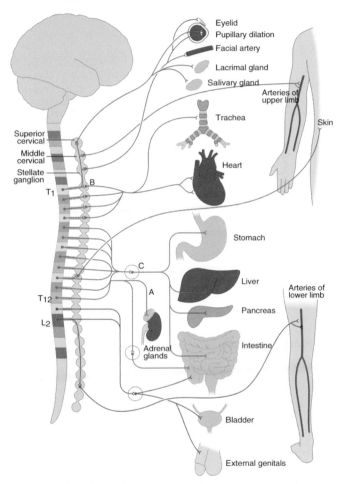

Efferents from the spinal cord to sympathetic effector organs. (**A**) Direct, one-neuron connections to the adrenal medulla. (**B**) Two-neuron pathways to the periphery and thoracic viscera, with synapses in paravertebral ganglia. (**C**) Two-neuron pathways to the abdominal and pelvic organs, with synapses in outlying ganglia.[37]

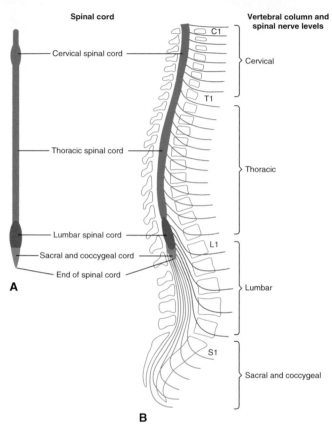

Spinal cord

Vertebral column and spinal nerve levels

C1

Cervical spinal cord — Cervical

T1

Thoracic spinal cord — Thoracic

Lumbar spinal cord —

Sacral and coccygeal cord —

End of spinal cord —

L1

A

Lumbar

S1

Sacral and coccygeal

B

Relationship of spinal cord segments to the vertebral column. (**A**) Anterior view of the spinal cord. (**B**) Spinal cord segment levels (neurologic levels) are indicated on the left. Vertebral levels and spinal nerves are indicated on the right. Spinal nerves are named for the vertebral level at which they exit the vertebral canal. The spinal cord ends at the L2 vertebral level. Because the spinal cord is significantly shorter than the vertebral column, only at C1 and C2 are the spinal cord segment levels and vertebral levels the same. The L2 to S5 nerve roots travel downward below the end of the spinal cord before exiting the vertebral canal. This collection of nerve roots inferior to the spinal cord within the bony canal is the cauda equina.[37]

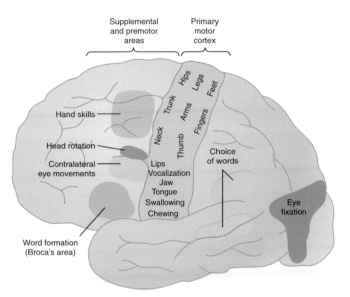

Representation of the different muscles of the body in the motor cortex, and location of other cortical areas responsible for specific types of motor movements.[26]

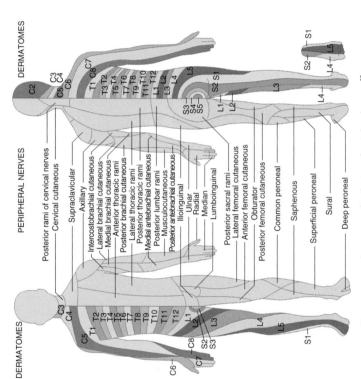

Dermatomes and cutaneous distribution of peripheral nerves.[37]

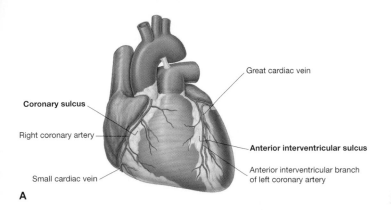

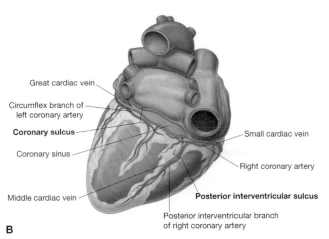

The heart. Anterior surface of the heart (**A**) and the diaphragmatic surface and base of the heart (**B**).[19]

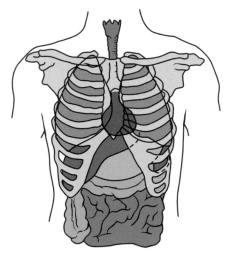

The relationship of the bony thorax and lungs to the abdominal contents (anterior view).[21]

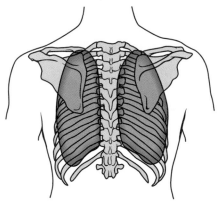

The relationship of the lungs to the bony thorax (posterior view).[21]

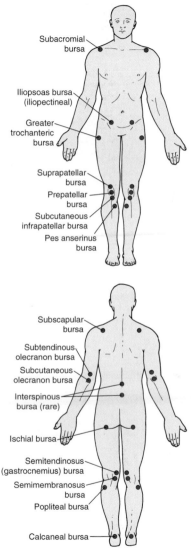

Sites of bursae. Bursae are fluid-filled sacs located at numerous points throughout the body. They are designed to provide a smooth gliding surface between bones, tendons, ligaments, muscles, and skin.[7]

Muscle Origin, Insertion, and Innervation[34]

Muscle	Origin (Proximal Attachment)	Insertion (Distal Attachment)	Action	Innervation
Pectoral Muscles				
Pectoralis major	Medial two thirds of clavicle; sternum; costal cartilages 1–6	Lateral lip of intertubercular groove (crest of greater tubercle) of humerus	Adduction and medial rotation of arm; flexion (clavicular fibers) and extension (sternocostal fibers) of arm	Medial and lateral pectoral nerves
Pectoralis minor	Ribs 3–5	Coracoid process of scapula	Depression of shoulder; downward rotation of scapula	Medial pectoral nerve
Sternocleidomastoid, Subclavius, Trapezius, and Latissimus Dorsi				
Sternocleidomastoid	Tendinous head from sternum; muscular head from medial third of clavicle	Mastoid process of skull	One muscle–flexion of neck toward same side (turns face to opposite side and brings ear of same side toward clavicle)	Accessory nerve
Subclavius	Rib 1	Undersurface of clavicle	Possibly depresses clavicle; maintains sternoclavicular joint	Nerve to subclavius
Trapezius	External occipital protuberance; ligamentum nuchae; spinous processes of seventh cervical and all thoracic vertebrae	Spine of scapula: acromion; lateral third of clavicle	Elevation of scapula (upper fibers); retraction of scapula (middle fibers); depression of scapula (inferior fibers); rotation of glenoid cavity upward	Accessory nerve (C3 and C4 sensory)
Latissimus dorsi	Spinous processes of lower six thoracic and all lumbar and sacral vertebrae; posterior part of iliac crest	Medial lip (crest of lesser tubercle) and floor of intertubercular groove of humerus	Extension, adduction, and medial rotation of arm	Thoracodorsal nerve
Levator Scapulae, Rhomboid Minor, and Rhomboid Major				
Levator scapulae	Transverse processes of upper four cervical vertebrae	Superior angle and upper part of medial border of scapula	Elevation of scapula	C3 and C4; dorsal scapular nerve

Muscle	Origin	Insertion	Action	Nerve
Rhomboid minor	Lower part of ligamentum nuchae; spinous processes of seventh cervical and first thoracic vertebrae	Medial border of scapula at base of spine	Elevation and retraction of scapula; downward rotation of glenoid cavity	Dorsal scapular nerve
Rhomboid major	Spinous processes of second to fifth thoracic vertebrae	Medial border of scapula below rhomboid minor	Elevation and retraction of scapula; downward rotation of glenoid cavity	Dorsal scapular nerve
Serratus Anterior				
Serratus anterior	Ribs 1–8 on anterolateral thoracic wall	Medial border of scapula; heaviest insertion to inferior angle	Protraction of scapula; upward rotation of glenoid cavity; holds medial border against thoracic wall	Long thoracic nerve
Deltoid				
Deltoid	Lateral third of clavicle; acromion; spine of scapula	Deltoid tuberosity on shaft of humerus	Abduction (middle fibers), flexion and medial rotation (anterior fibers), and extension and lateral rotation (posterior fibers) of arm	Axillary nerve
Supraspinatus, Infraspinatus, Teres Minor, Teres Major, and Subscapularis				
Supraspinatus	Supraspinous fossa of scapula	Greater tubercle of humerus	Abduction of arm	Suprascapular nerve
Infraspinatus	Infraspinous fossa of scapula	Greater tubercle of humerus below supraspinatus	Lateral rotation of arm	Suprascapular nerve
Teres minor	Upper two thirds of lateral border of scapula	Greater tubercle of humerus below infraspinatus	Lateral rotation of arm	Axillary nerve
Teres major	Inferior angle of scapula	Medial lip of intertubercular groove of humerus	Adduction, medial rotation, and extension of arm	Lower subscapular nerve
Subscapularis	Subscapular fossa of scapula	Lesser tubercle and crest of humerus	Medial rotation of arm	Upper and lower subscapular nerves
Biceps Brachii				
Biceps brachii	Short head—tip of coracoid process of scapula	Radial tuberosity and bicipital aponeurosis into fascia of forearm	Flexion and supination of forearm; flexion of arm	Musculocutaneous nerve

Continued

Muscle	Origin (Proximal Attachment)	Insertion (Distal Attachment)	Action	Innervation
Coracobrachialis and Brachialis				
Coracobrachialis	Coracoid process of scapula	Anteromedial surface of midshaft of humerus	Flexion and adduction of arm	Musculocutaneous nerve
Brachialis	Lower half of anterior surface of humerus; intermuscular septa	Ulnar tuberosity	Flexion of forearm	Musculocutaneous nerve (lateral side may receive twig from radial nerve)
Triceps Brachii and Anconeus				
Triceps brachii	Long head—infraglenoid tubercle of scapula	Proximal end of olecranon of ulna	Extension of forearm; extension of arm (long head)	Radial nerve
	Lateral head—posterior surface of humerus above and lateral to groove of radial nerve and lateral intermuscular septum			
	Medial head—posterior surface of humerus below and medial to groove of radial nerve and both intermuscular septa			
Anconeus	Lateral epicondyle of humerus	Lateral side of olecranon of ulna	Extension of forearm	Radial nerve
Superficial Muscles				
Pronator teres	Medial epicondyle of humerus; coronoid process of ulna	Lateral surface of mid-shaft of radius	Pronation of forearm (and hand)	Median nerve
Palmaris longus	Medial epicondyle of humerus (common flexor tendon)	Palmar aponeurosis	Flexion of hand	Median nerve
Flexor carpi radialis	Medial epicondyle of humerus (common flexor tendon)	Base of second metacarpal and possibly third metacarpal	Flexion and abduction (radial deviation) of hand	Median nerve

Muscle	Origin	Insertion	Action	Nerve
Flexor carpi ulnaris	Medial epicondyle of humerus (common flexor tendon); proximal two thirds of posterior surface of ulna	Pisiform bone	Flexion and adduction (ulnar deviation) of hand	Ulnar nerve
Intermediate Muscle				
Flexor digitorum superficialis	Medial epicondyle of humerus (common flexor tendon); medial aspect of coronoid process of ulna; proximal half of radius distal to radial tuberosity	Base of middle phalanx of each of four fingers (medial four digits)	Flexion of middle phalanx of each of four fingers (medial four digits); with continued action flexion of each proximal phalanx; aids in flexion of hand	Median nerve
Deep Muscles				
Flexor digitorum profundus	Anterior and medial surfaces of proximal two thirds of ulna; interosseous membrane; aponeurosis of flexor carpi ulnaris	Distal phalanx of each of four fingers (medial four digits)	Flexion of distal phalanx of each of four fingers (medial four digits); with continued action flexion of the middle and proximal phalanges; aids in flexion of hand	Median and ulnar nerves
Flexor pollicis longus	Anterior surface of middle half of radius; adjacent interosseous membrane	Distal phalanx of thumb	Flexion of distal phalanx of thumb	Median nerve
Pronator quadratus	Distal fourth of ulna	Distal part of radius	Pronation of forearm (and hand)	Median nerve
Superficial Muscles of the Extensor Forearm				
Brachioradialis	Lateral supracondylar ridge of humerus; intermuscular septum of arm	Lateral side of distal end of radius	Flexion of forearm	Radial nerve
Extensor carpi radialis longus	Lateral supracondylar ridge and lateral epicondyle of humerus (common extensor tendon); intermuscular septum	Base of second metacarpal	Extension and abduction (radial deviation) of hand	Radial nerve

Continued

Muscle	Origin (Proximal Attachment)	Insertion (Distal Attachment)	Action	Innervation
Extensor carpi radialis brevis	Lateral epicondyle of humerus (common extensor tendon); intermuscular septum; antebrachial fascia	Base of third metacarpal	Extension of hand	Radial nerve
Extensor digitorum	Lateral epicondyle of humerus; intermuscular septum; antebrachial fascia	Middle and distal phalanges of each of four fingers (medial four digits)	Extension of each of four fingers (medial four digits)	Radial nerve
Extensor digiti minimi	Lateral epicondyle of humerus (common extensor tendon)	Middle and distal phalanges of little finger	Extension and abduction of little finger	Radial nerve
Extensor carpi ulnaris	Lateral epicondyle of humerus (common extensor tendon); proximal part of ulna	Base of fifth metacarpal	Extension and adduction (ulnar deviation) of hand	Radial nerve
Deep Muscles of the Extensor Forearm				
Supinator	Posterolateral surface of ulna below radial notch; lateral epicondyle; radial collateral and annular ligaments	Proximal shaft of radius	Supination of forearm (and hand)	Radial nerve
Abductor pollicis longus	Posterior surface of ulna and radius; interosseous membrane	Base of first metacarpal	Abduction and extension of thumb	Radial nerve
Extensor pollicis brevis	Posterior surface of radius; interosseous membrane	Proximal phalanx of thumb	Extension of proximal phalanx of thumb	Radial nerve
Extensor pollicis longus	Posterior surface of middle third of ulna; interosseous membrane	Distal phalanx of thumb	Extension of distal phalanx of thumb	Radial nerve
Extensor indicis	Posterior surface of ulna; interosseous membrane	Extensor expansion of index finger	Extension of index finger	Radial nerve

Lumbricals			
Lumbricals (4)	Tendons of flexor digitorum profundus	Extensor expansion of medial four digits	Extension of interphalangeal joints of medial four digits; flexion of metacarpophalangeal joints	Median nerve (lateral two); ulnar nerve (medial two)

Muscles of the Thumb			
Abductor pollicis brevis	Flexor retinaculum; scaphoid and trapezium	Base of proximal phalanx of thumb	Abduction of thumb	Median nerve
Opponens pollicis	Flexor retinaculum; trapezium	First metacarpal	Opposition of thumb	Median nerve
Flexor pollicis brevis	Superficial head—flexor retinaculum (and possibly trapezium) Deep head—trapezoid and capitate	Base of proximal phalanx of thumb	Flexion of thumb; aids in opposition and adduction	Median nerve (superficial head); ulnar nerve (deep head)
Adductor pollicis	Transverse head—third metacarpal Oblique head—bases of first three metacarpals, and capitate, trapezoid, and trapezium	Base of proximal phalanx of thumb	Adduction and flexion of thumb	Ulnar nerve

Muscles of the Little Finger			
Palmaris brevis	Palmar aponeurosis, medial border	Skin on ulnar side of hand	Stabilization of skin of palm for gripping	Ulnar nerve
Abductor digiti minimi	Pisiform	Base of proximal phalanx of little finger	Abduction of little finger	Ulnar nerve
Flexor digiti minimi brevis	Flexor retinaculum; hook of hamate	Proximal phalanx of little finger	Flexion of little finger	Ulnar nerve
Opponens digiti minimi	Flexor retinaculum; hook of hamate	Fifth metacarpal	Opposition of little finger to thumb	Ulnar nerve

Continued

Muscle	Origin (Proximal Attachment)	Insertion (Distal Attachment)	Action	Innervation
Interossei				
Palmar interossei (3)	Shaft of metacarpal—one to each of index, ring, and little fingers	Extensor expansion of finger of origin	Adduction of the respective finger; index, ring, and little fingers; flexion of metacarpophalangeal joints; extension of interphalangeal joints	Ulnar nerve
Dorsal interossei (4)	Adjacent surfaces of two metacarpals	No. 1—proximal phalanx on radial side of index finger Nos. 2, 3, and 4—proximal phalanx on radial side of middle, ulnar side of ring fingers, respectively, and extensor expansion	Abduction of index, middle, and ring fingers; flexion of metacarpophalangeal joints; extension of interphalangeal joints (depending on insertion, No. 1 may not extend interphalangeal joints)	Ulnar nerve
Splenius Muscles				
Splenius capitis	Ligamentum nuchae; spinous processes of seventh cervical and first three or four thoracic vertebrae	Mastoid process and occipital bone of skull	Rotation of head and cervical vertebral column to same side; bilateral action—extension of head	Posterior rami of middle cervical spinal nerves
Splenius cervicis	Spinous processes of third to sixth thoracic vertebrae	Transverse processes of upper two to four cervical vertebrae	Rotation of head and cervical vertebral column to same side; bilateral action—extension of head and vertebral column	Posterior rami of lower cervical spinal nerves
Serratus Posterior Muscles				
Serratus posterior superior	Ligamentum nuchae; spinous processes of seventh cervical and upper two or three thoracic vertebrae	Upper ribs, usually 2-5	Elevation of ribs	Anterior rami of upper three or four thoracic spinal nerves (intercostals)

Serratus posterior inferior	Spinous processes of lower two thoracic and upper two lumbar vertebrae	Lower three or four ribs	Pulls lower ribs inferiorly	Anterior rami of lower thoracic (ninth to twelfth) spinal nerves (intercostals)
Erector Spinae Muscles				
Erector spinae (component muscles listed below in anatomical order)	Common tendon of origin; posterior surface of sacrum, iliac crest, spinous processes of lumbar and last two thoracic vertebrae (specific origins given below)	As described for each muscle	Bilateral action—extension of vertebral column Unilateral action—bend vertebral column toward same side (lateral flexion) (Note: This is action for all muscles of this group)	Posterior rami of spinal nerves in area of muscle (Note: this is innervation for all muscles of this group)
Iliocostalis lumborum	Iliac crest; sacrum	Lower borders of lower six or seven ribs	See erector spinae	See erector spinae
Iliocostalis thoracis	Upper borders of lower six or seven ribs	Lower borders of upper six or seven ribs	See erector spinae	See erector spinae
Iliocostalis cervicis	Angles of upper six ribs	Transverse processes of fourth to sixth cervical vertebrae	See erector spinae	See erector spinae
Longissimus thoracis	Intermediate part of common tendon	Lower nine or ten ribs and adjacent transverse processes of vertebrae	See erector spinae	See erector spinae
Longissimus cervicis	Transverse processes of upper four to six thoracic vertebrae	Transverse process of second to sixth cervical vertebrae	See erector spinae	See erector spinae
Longissimus capitis	Tendons of origin of longissimus cervicis; articular processes of lower four cervical vertebrae	Mastoid process of skull	See erector spinae	See erector spinae
Spinalis thoracis	Spinous process of lower two thoracic and upper two lumbar vertebrae	Spinous processes of upper thoracic vertebrae (varies from four to eight)	See erector spinae	See erector spinae

Continued

Muscle	Origin (Proximal Attachment)	Insertion (Distal Attachment)	Action	Innervation
Spinalis cervicis	Ligamentum nuchae; spinous processes of seventh cervical and upper one or two thoracic vertebrae	Spinous process of axis (and possibly third and fourth cervical vertebrae)	See erector spinae	See erector spinae
Spinalis capitis	(Considered as the medial part of semispinalis capitis)			
Transversospinales Muscles				
Semispinalis thoracis	Transverse processes of lower six thoracic vertebrae	Spinous processes of lower two cervical and upper four thoracic vertebrae	Extension of vertebral column	Posterior rami of cervical and thoracic spinal nerves
Semispinalis cervicis	Transverse processes of upper five or six thoracic vertebrae	Spinous processes of second to fifth cervical vertebrae	Extension of vertebral column	Posterior rami of cervical and thoracic spinal nerves
Semispinalis capitis	Transverse processes of upper six or seven thoracic vertebrae; articular processes of lower three cervical vertebrae	Occipital bone (between superior and inferior nuchal lines)	Extension of head	Posterior rami of cervical and thoracic spinal nerves
Multifidus	Sacrum and posterior superior iliac spine; mammillary processes of lumbar vertebrae; transverse processes of thoracic vertebrae; articular processes of lower cervical vertebrae	Spinous processes of lumbar through second cervical vertebrae: Fascicles span two to four segments of the column	Extension, lateral flexion, and rotation (to opposite side) of the vertebral column	Posterior rami of spinal nerves
Rotatores	Sacrum and transverse processes of lumbar through lower cervical vertebrae	Spinous processes of lumbar through second cervical vertebrae: Fascicles span one to two segments of the column	Rotation (to opposite side) and extension of vertebral column	Posterior rami of spinal nerves

Muscle	Origin	Insertion	Action	Nerve
Segmental Muscles				
Interspinales	Spinous processes of vertebrae (absent in much of thoracic region)	Spinous processes of vertebra (span between adjacent vertebrae)	Extension of vertebral column	Posterior rami of cervical spinal nerves
Intertransversarii	Transverse processes of vertebrae (absent in much of thoracic region)	Transverse processes of vertebrae (span between adjacent vertebrae)	Lateral flexion of vertebral column (unilateral action)	Posterior and anterior rami of spinal nerves
Suboccipital and Deep Neck Muscles				
Obliquus capitis inferior	Spinous process of axis	Transverse process of atlas	Rotation of atlas (turn head to same side)	Posterior ramus of C1
Obliquus capitis superior	Transverse process of atlas	Occipital bone	Extension and lateral bending of head	Posterior ramus of C1
Rectus capitis posterior major	Spinous process of axis	Occipital bone	Extension of head; rotation of head to same side	Posterior ramus of C1
Rectus capitis posterior minor	Posterior tubercle of atlas	Occipital bone	Extension of head	Posterior ramus of C1
Longus colli	Bodies of first to third thoracic vertebrae; transverse processes of third to fifth cervical vertebrae; bodies of upper three thoracic and lower three cervical vertebrae	Transverse processes of fifth and sixth cervical vertebrae; anterior surface of atlas; bodies of second to fourth cervical vertebrae (respectively with listed origins)	Flexion; possibly lateral flexion of neck	Anterior rami of C2-C6
Longus capitis	Transverse processes of third to sixth cervical vertebrae	Occipital bone	Flexion of head and upper cervical vertebrae	Anterior rami of C1-C3
Rectus capitis anterior	Lateral mass of atlas	Occipital bone	Stabilization of atlanto-occipital joint; flexion of head	Anterior rami of C1 and C2
Rectus capitis lateralis	Transverse process of atlas	Occipital bone	Stabilization of atlanto-occipital joint; lateral flexion of head	Anterior rami of C1 and C2

Continued

Muscle	Origin (Proximal Attachment)	Insertion (Distal Attachment)	Action	Innervation
Anterior Muscles of the Thigh				
Sartorius	Anterior superior iliac spine	Medial surface—proximal end of tibia just distal to tibial tuberosity	Flexion, abduction, and lateral rotation of thigh; flexion of leg	Femoral nerve
Tensor fasciae latae	Iliac crest posterior to anterior superior iliac spine	Iliotibial tract	Flexion, medial rotation, and abduction of thigh	Superior gluteal nerve
Quadriceps Femoris				
Rectus femoris	Anterior inferior iliac spine; ilium above acetabulum	Patella and through patellar ligament to tibial tuberosity	Extension of leg; flexion of thigh	Femoral nerve
Vastus medialis	Medial lip of linea aspera; lower part of intertrochanteric line	Patella and through patellar ligament to tibial tuberosity	Extension of leg	Femoral nerve
Vastus lateralis	Lateral lip of linea aspera of femur; limited origin from intertrochanteric line	Patella and through patellar ligament to tibial tuberosity	Extension of leg	Femoral nerve
Vastus intermedius	Anterior and lateral surfaces of femur	Patella and through patellar ligament to tibial tuberosity	Extension of leg	Femoral nerve
Articularis genus	Distal part of anterior surface of femur	Synovial membrane of knee joint	Pulls synovial membrane of knee proximally during extension of leg	Femoral nerve (nerve to vastus intermedius)
Iliopsoas				
Psoas major	Bodies and transverse processes of lumbar vertebrae (and possibly last thoracic vertebra)	Lesser trochanter of femur	Flexion of thigh; slight adduction of thigh of free limb	Second to fourth lumbar nerves
Iliacus	Iliac fossa	Lesser trochanter (with psoas major) of femur	Flexion of thigh; slight adduction of thigh of free limb	Femoral nerve
Psoas minor	Twelfth thoracic and first lumbar vertebrae	Superior ramus of pubis	Upward rotation of pelvis	First or second lumbar nerve (or both)

	Origin	Insertion	Action	Nerve
Pectineus	Superior ramus of pubis	Femur just distal to lesser trochanter	Flexion and adduction of thigh	Femoral nerve; possibly obturator and/or accessory obturator nerve
Adductor Group of Muscles				
Adductor longus	Pubic tubercle	Medial lip of linea aspera of femur	Adduction and flexion of thigh	Obturator nerve
Gracilis	Inferior ramus of pubis; ramus of ischium	Medial surface—proximal end of tibia just distal to medial condyle	Adduction of thigh; flexion of leg; medial rotation of flexed leg	Obturator nerve
Adductor brevis	Body and inferior ramus of pubis	Pectineal line; proximal part of linea aspera of femur	Adduction and flexion of thigh	Obturator nerve
Adductor magnus	Inferior ramus of pubis; ramus of ischium; ischial tuberosity	Linea aspera (anterior fibers); adductor tubercle of femur (posterior fibers)	Adduction of thigh; flexion of thigh (anterior fibers); extension of thigh (posterior fibers)	Obturator nerve (anterior fibers); sciatic nerve (posterior fibers)
Obturator externus	Obturator membrane; bone around obturator foramen on external surface of pelvis	Trochanteric fossa of femur	Lateral rotation of thigh	Obturator nerve
Muscles of the Gluteal Region				
Gluteus maximus	Lateral surface of ilium behind posterior gluteal line; posterior sacroiliac and sacrotuberous ligaments; posterior surface of sacrum	Iliotibial tract; gluteal tuberosity of femur	Extension, lateral rotation, abduction (upper fibers), and adduction (lower fibers) of thigh	Inferior gluteal nerve
Gluteus medius	Lateral surface of ilium between anterior and posterior gluteal lines	Greater trochanter of femur	Abduction of thigh; medial rotation and flexion (anterior fibers) and lateral rotation and extension (posterior fibers) of thigh	Superior gluteal nerve

Continued

Muscle	Origin (Proximal Attachment)	Insertion (Distal Attachment)	Action	Innervation
Gluteus minimus	Lateral surface of ilium between anterior and inferior gluteal lines	Greater trochanter of femur	Abduction of thigh; medial rotation and flexion of thigh	Superior gluteal nerve
Piriformis	Sacrum (anterior surface)	Greater trochanter of femur	Lateral rotation of thigh; abduction of thigh when thigh is flexed	S1 and S2
Obturator internus	Obturator membrane; bone around obturator foramen on internal surface of pelvis	Medial surface of greater trochanter above trochanteric fossa of femur	Lateral rotation of thigh; abduction of thigh when thigh is flexed	Nerve to obturator internus
Superior gemellus	Ischial spine	Superior border of obturator internus tendon	Lateral rotation of thigh; abduction of thigh when thigh is flexed	Nerve to obturator internus
Inferior gemellus	Ischial tuberosity	Inferior border of obturator internus tendon	Lateral rotation of thigh; abduction of thigh when thigh is flexed	Nerve to quadratus femoris
Quadratus femoris	Ischial tuberosity	Posterior surface of femur between greater and lesser trochanters	Lateral rotation and adduction of thigh	Nerve to quadratus femoris
Posterior Muscles of the Thigh				
Semitendinosus	Ischial tuberosity	Medial surface of proximal end of tibia	Extension of thigh; flexion of leg; medial rotation of flexed leg	Sciatic nerve—tibial part
Semimembranosus	Ischial tuberosity	Medial condyle of tibia	Extension of thigh; flexion of leg; medial rotation of flexed leg	Sciatic nerve—tibial part
Biceps femoris	Long head—ischial tuberosity Short head—linea aspera of femur and lateral intermuscular septum	Head of fibula	Extension of thigh (long head); flexion of leg (long head); lateral rotation of flexed leg	Sciatic nerve—tibial part to long head; common fibular part to short head
Superficial Muscles of the Calf				
Gastrocnemius	Posterior surface of femur just proximal to medial and lateral condyles	Calcaneus through calcaneal tendon	Plantar flexion of foot: flexion of leg of free limb	Tibial nerve

Muscle	Origin	Insertion	Action	Nerve
Soleus	Soleal (or popliteal) line; posterior surface of upper third and medial border of middle third of tibia; proximal third of posterior surface of fibula	Calcaneus through calcaneal tendon	Plantar flexion of foot	Tibial nerve
Plantaris	Lateral epicondyle of femur	Calcaneus (anteromedial to calcaneal tendon)	Weak plantar flexion of foot; weak flexion of leg	Tibial nerve
Deep Muscles of the Calf				
Popliteus	Lateral condyle of femur	Proximal third of posterior aspect of tibia (proximal to soleal line)	Medial rotation of leg on femur; lateral rotation of femur on leg	Tibial nerve
Flexor hallucis longus	Middle half of posterior surface of fibula	Distal phalanx of big toe	Flexion of big toe; weak plantar flexion of foot	Tibial nerve
Flexor digitorum longus	Middle third of posterior surface of tibia	Distal phalanges of lateral four toes	Flexion of distal phalanges of lateral four toes; weak plantar flexion and inversion of foot	Tibial nerve
Tibialis posterior	Proximal two thirds of posterior surface of tibia; proximal two thirds of fibula; interosseous membrane	Navicular; cuneiforms; cuboid; bases of second to fourth metatarsals	Adduct front of foot; inversion and plantar flexion of foot	Tibial nerve
Lateral Muscles of the Leg				
Fibularis longus	Proximal two thirds of lateral surface of fibula; adjacent fascia and intermuscular septa	Base of first metatarsal; medial cuneiform	Eversion and weak plantar flexion of foot	Superficial fibular nerve (and often a branch from common or deep fibular nerve)
Fibularis brevis	Distal two thirds of lateral surface of fibula; adjacent intermuscular septa	Dorsal surface of base of fifth metatarsal	Eversion and weak plantar flexion of foot	Superficial fibular nerve

Continued

Muscle	Origin (Proximal Attachment)	Insertion (Distal Attachment)	Action	Innervation
Anterior Muscles of the Leg				
Extensor digitorum longus	Lateral condyle of tibia; proximal three fourths of anterior surface of fibula; interosseous membrane and crural fascia	Middle and distal phalanges of lateral four toes	Extension of lateral four toes; dorsiflexion and eversion of foot	Deep fibular nerve
Fibularis tertius	Fibula in common with lower fibers of extensor digitorum longus	Dorsal surface of base of fifth metatarsal	Dorsiflexion and eversion of foot	Deep fibular nerve
Extensor hallucis longus	Middle third of anterior surface of fibula; interosseous membrane	Distal phalanx of big toe	Extension of big toe; dorsiflexion and inversion of foot	Deep fibular nerve
Tibialis anterior	Lateral condyle of tibia; proximal two thirds of lateral surface of tibia; interosseous membrane; and deep fascia of leg	Medial cuneiform; base of first metatarsal	Inversion and dorsiflexion of foot	Deep fibular nerve
Plantar Muscles—Superficial Layer				
Abductor hallucis	Medial process of calcaneal tuberosity; flexor retinaculum; medial intermuscular septum	Proximal phalanx of big toe (tibial side of flexor surface)	Flexion and abduction of big toe at metatarsophalangeal joint	Medial plantar nerve
Flexor digitorum brevis	Medial process of calcaneal tuberosity; medial and lateral intermuscular septa	Middle phalanges of lateral four toes	Flexion of middle phalanges of lateral four toes	Medial plantar nerve
Abductor digiti minimi	Lateral process of calcaneal tuberosity; medial process (small area); intervening surface of calcaneus	Proximal phalanx of little toe (lateral side)	Flexion and abduction of little toe	Lateral plantar nerve
Plantar Muscles—Second Layer				
Quadratus plantae	Medial and lateral sides of plantar surface of calcaneus (distal to calcaneal tuberosity)	Lateral and posterior margin of tendon of flexor digitorum longus	Aids in flexion of lateral four toes by modifying pull of flexor digitorum longus tendon	Lateral plantar nerve

Muscle	Proximal Attachment	Distal Attachment	Action	Innervation
Lumbricals	Flexor digitorum longus tendons	Expansions of extensor tendons of lateral four toes	Flexion of metatarsophalangeal joints; possible extension of interphalangeal joints	Medial plantar nerve to first lumbrical; lateral plantar nerve to second, third, and fourth lumbricals
Plantar Muscles—Third Layer				
Flexor hallucis brevis	Cuboid bone; lateral cuneiform bone; tendon of tibialis posterior muscle	Medial and lateral sides of proximal phalanx of big toe	Flexion of proximal phalanx of big toe	Medial plantar nerve
Adductor hallucis	Oblique head—bases of second to fourth metatarsals; sheath of fibularis longus tendon. Transverse head—capsules of third to fifth metatarsophalangeal joints; associated deep transverse metatarsal ligaments	Base of proximal phalanx of big toe	Adduction and flexion of big toe	Lateral plantar nerve
Flexor digiti minimi brevis	Base of fifth metatarsal	Base of proximal phalanx of little toe (plantar surface)	Flexion of proximal phalanx of little toe	Lateral plantar nerve
Plantar Muscles—Deep Layer				
Plantar interossei	Medial side of third through fifth metatarsals	Medial side of proximal phalanges of same toes	Adduction of toes	Lateral plantar nerve
Dorsal interossei	Adjacent sides of metatarsals	Proximal phalanges: No. 1 to medial side of second toe; Nos. 2, 3, and 4 to lateral side of correspondingly numbered toes	Abduction of toes	Lateral plantar nerve
Dorsal Muscles				
Extensor digitorum brevis	Calcaneus (dorsal surface)	Extensor digitorum longus tendons to second to fourth toes	Extension of second to fourth toes	Deep fibular nerve

Continued

Muscle	Origin (Proximal Attachment)	Insertion (Distal Attachment)	Action	Innervation
Extensor hallucis brevis (often considered medial part of extensor digitorum brevis)	Calcaneus (dorsal surface)	Base of proximal phalanx of big toe	Extension of big toe	Deep fibular nerve
Muscles of Mastication				
Masseter	Zygomatic arch	Ramus and angle of mandible (lateral surface)	Elevation of mandible; superficial head may aid in protrusion of mandible	Trigeminal nerve—mandibular division
Temporalis	Lateral surface of skull (temporal fossa)	Coronoid process and anterior part of ramus of mandible (medial surface)	Elevation of mandible; retrusion of mandible (posterior fibers)	Trigeminal nerve—mandibular division
Lateral pterygoid	Lateral surface of lateral pterygoid plate of sphenoid bone; sphenoid bone (greater wing)	Neck of mandible, and capsule and disc of temporomandibular joint	Protrusion of mandible	Trigeminal nerve—mandibular division
Medial pterygoid	Medial surface of lateral pterygoid plate of sphenoid bone; maxillary tuberosity	Ramus and angle of mandible (medial surface)	Elevation of mandible	Trigeminal nerve—mandibular division
Muscles of the Neck				
Sternocleidomastoid	Sternum and medial third of clavicle	Mastoid process of temporal bone	Both muscles—flexion of head and neck One muscle—lateral flexion (turns face to opposite side)	Accessory nerve (motor); C2 and C3 (sensory)
Sternohyoid	Sternum (posterior surface)	Hyoid bone	Depression and/or fixation of hyoid bone	Anterior rami of first three cervical spinal nerves through ansa cervicalis
Sternothyroid	Sternum (posterior surface)	Thyroid cartilage	Depression and/or fixation of thyroid cartilage	Anterior rami of first three cervical spinal nerves through ansa cervicalis

Muscle	Origin	Insertion	Action	Innervation
Thyrohyoid	Thyroid cartilage	Hyoid bone	Depression and/or stabilization of hyoid bone; if hyoid bone is fixed, elevation of thyroid cartilage	Anterior ramus of C1 by way of hypoglossal nerve
Omohyoid	Superior border of scapula	Hyoid bone	Depression and/or fixation of hyoid bone	Anterior rami of first three cervical spinal nerves through ansa cervicalis
Anterior scalene	Transverse processes of third to sixth cervical vertebrae	First rib	Fixation of elevation of first rib during inhalation — With rib fixed—lateral flexion of neck	Anterior rami of cervical spinal nerves at origin of muscle
Middle scalene	Transverse processes of lower five or six cervical vertebrae (possibly the atlas)	First rib	Fixation or elevation of first rib during inhalation — With rib fixed—lateral flexion of neck	Anterior rami of cervical spinal nerves at origin of muscle
Posterior scalene	Transverse processes of fourth to sixth cervical vertebrae	Second rib	Fixation or elevation of second rib — With rib fixed—lateral flexion of neck	Anterior rami of cervical spinal nerves at origin of muscle
External and Internal Intercostal Muscles				
External intercostals	Lower border of rib (11 pairs)	Upper border of rib below origin	Maintains intercostal space; variable reports of involvement in inspiration/expiration	Intercostal nerves
Internal intercostals	Lower border of rib (11 pairs)	Upper border of rib below origin	Maintains intercostal space; variable reports on involvement in inspiration/expiration	Intercostal nerves
Diaphragm				
Diaphragm	Deep surface of xiphoid process; lower ribs anteriorly and laterally; bodies of upper lumbar vertebrae as crura of diaphragm; fascia over psoas major and quadratus lumborum	Central tendon of diaphragm	Depression of central tendon to increase vertical dimension of thoracic cavity	Phrenic nerve (C3, C4, C5)

Continued

Muscle	Origin (Proximal Attachment)	Insertion (Distal Attachment)	Action	Innervation
Muscles of the Abdominal Wall				
External oblique	Lower six ribs	Anterior part of iliac crest; pubis; aponeurosis into linea alba	With internal oblique and transversus abdominis—compression of abdominal cavity; flexion and rotation of trunk	Lower intercostal nerves; iliohypogastric and ilioinguinal nerves
Internal oblique	Iliopsoas fascia and inguinal ligament; anterior part of iliac crest; thoracolumbar fascia	Aponeurosis into linea alba; lower ribs	Compression of abdominal cavity; flexion and rotation of trunk	Lower intercostal nerves; iliohypogastric and ilioinguinal nerves
Transversus abdominis	Thoracolumbar fascia; tips of lower six ribs; anterior part of iliac crest; iliopsoas fascia and inguinal ligament	Aponeurosis into linea alba	Compression of abdominal cavity	Lower intercostal nerves; iliohypogastric and ilioinguinal nerves
Rectus abdominis	Pubic crest; ligaments of pubic symphysis	Xiphoid process; ribs 5–7	Flexion of trunk	Lower intercostal nerves
Quadratus Lumborum				
Quadratus lumborum	Medial part of iliac crest	Rib 12; lower lumbar vertebrae	Lateral flexion of vertebral column; fixes last rib to form stable base for contraction of diaphragm	Branches from T12 and L1–L3
Pelvic Diaphragm				
Levator ani (component parts: puborectalis; pubococcygeus; and iliococcygeus)	Pubis; ischial spine; fascia between bony origins	Coccyx; midline around pelvic organs and with muscle of opposite side	Support of pelvic viscera, particularly during increased abdominal pressure	Branches from S3 and S4
Ischiococcygeus (coccygeus)	Ischial spine	Lower sacrum; upper coccyx	Pulls coccyx anteriorly; support of pelvic viscera	Branches from S4 and S5

Anatomical Directional Terms[37]

Term	Definition	Antonym	Definition of Antonym
Superior	Above another part	Inferior	Below another part
Rostral	Toward the head	Caudal	Toward the tail or coccyx
Anterior or ventral	Toward the front	Posterior or dorsal	Toward the back
Medial	Toward the midline	Lateral	Farther from the midline
Proximal	Nearest the point of origin	Distal	Farther from the point of origin
Ipsilateral	On the same side of the body	Contralateral	On the opposite side of the body

Cranial Nerve Function[37]

#	Name	Function
I	Olfactory	Smell
II	Optic	Vision
III	Oculomotor	Moves eyes up, down, medially; raises upper eyelid; constricts pupil
IV	Trochlear	Moves eye medially and down
V	Trigeminal	Facial sensation, chewing, sensation from temporomandibular joint
VI	Abducens	Abducts eye
VII	Facial	Facial expression, closes eyes, tears, salivation, and taste
VIII	Acoustic	Sensation of head position relative to gravity and head movement; hearing
IX	Glossopharyngeal	Swallowing, salivation, and taste
X	Vagus	Regulates viscera, swallowing, speech, and taste
XI	Accessory	Elevates shoulders, turns head
XII	Hypoglossal	Moves tongue

Examination

Patient Examination

Sample/Evaluation Sequence[4]

Review of medical history/patient profile

↓

History/interview
What questions to include/exclude?

↓

Presenting complaints/functional limitations

↓

Review relevant medical history

↓

Review of systems
(General health)

↓

Review of systems
(Specific systems)
Cardiovascular/pulmonary/gastrointestinal/urogenital/
psychological/endocrine/nervous system/integumentary

↓

Physical examination
What exams, tests or measures to include or exclude?
Vital signs/height/weight/upper or lower quarter
examinations/systems review

↓

Evaluate data
Does the patient need a referral or consultation?

↓

Treat/treat and refer/refer only

History and Review of Systems[24]

The first step in making a diagnosis is to confirm (or rule out) the need for physical therapy intervention. Use this screening checklist to answer these questions:

- Is this an appropriate physical therapy referral?
- Is there a problem that does not fall into one of the four categories of conditions outlined by the Guide (musculoskeletal, neuromuscular, cardiovascular/pulmonary, and integumentary)?
- Are there any red-flag histories, red-flag risk factors, or cluster of red-flag signs and/or symptoms?
- And always ask: Were you examined by a (your) doctor?

This quick screening examination, as part of the overall physical therapy evaluation, includes each of the following components:

PAST MEDICAL HISTORY

Previous history of:

Cardiovascular disease
Cancer
Diabetes
Infection (any kind)
Pulmonary disease
Recent surgery
Trauma
Tuberculosis

For women: pregnancy, birth, miscarriage, abortion, and other reproductive history

Psychosocial screen (orientation [person, place, time]; anxiety, depression, panic disorder; recent travel overseas; occupational/environmental exposure)

Medications

RISK-FACTOR ASSESSMENT

Substance use/abuse
Age
Body mass index (BMI)
Gender
Race/ethnicity
Tobacco use
Overseas travel

Alcohol use/abuse
Occupation
Domestic violence
Hysterectomy/oophorectomy
Sedentary lifestyle
Exposure to radiation
Multiple sexual partners

CLINICAL PRESENTATION

General Survey	Upper Quadrant Exam	Lower Quadrant Exam
Level of consciousness Mental and emotional status Vision and hearing Speech General appearance Nutritional status Level of self-care Body size, type, and BMI Obvious deformities Muscle atrophy Body and breath odors Posture Movement patterns and gait Use of assistive devices or mobility aids Balance and coordination Inspect skin, hair, and nails Vital signs	Lymph node palpation Head and neck Cranial nerves Upper limbs: • Muscle tone and strength • Joint range of motion • Reflexes • Coordination • Motor and sensory function • Vascular assessment Chest and back (heart and lungs): • Inspection • Palpation • Auscultation Clinical breast examination (CBE)	Lymph node palpation Lower limbs: • Muscle tone and strength • Joint range of motion • Reflexes • Coordination • Motor and sensory function • Vascular assessment Abdomen: • Inspection • Auscultation • Palpation

Also note the following systems:
Integumentary
Musculoskeletal
Neuromuscular
Cardiopulmonary
Genitourinary

ASSOCIATED SIGNS AND SYMPTOMS

Always ask: Are there symptoms of any kind anywhere else in your body? If no, follow up with:

Have you had any (check all that apply):

☐ Blood in urine, stool, vomit, sputum/mucus
☐ Changes in bowel or bladder
☐ Confusion
☐ Cough
☐ Difficulty chewing/swallowing/speaking
☐ Dizziness, fainting, blackouts
☐ Dribbling or leaking urine
☐ Fever, chills, sweats (day or night)
☐ Headaches
☐ Heart palpitations or fluttering
☐ Joint pain
☐ Memory loss

☐ Nausea, vomiting, loss of appetite
☐ Numbness or tingling
☐ Problems seeing or hearing
☐ Skin rash or other changes
☐ Sudden weakness
☐ Swelling or lumps anywhere
☐ Trouble breathing
☐ Trouble sleeping
☐ Throbbing sensation/pain in belly or anywhere else
☐ Unusual fatigue, drowsiness

REVIEW OF SYSTEMS

When conducting a general review of systems, look for a cluster of signs and symptoms* to identify the possible involvement of one or more system(s). Ask the client about the presence of any other problems anywhere else in the body. Depending on the client's answer, you may want to prompt them about any of the following common signs and symptoms associated with each system:

General Questions
- Fever, chills, sweating (constitutional symptoms)
- Appetite loss, nausea, vomiting (constitutional symptoms)
- Fatigue, malaise, weakness (constitutional symptoms)
- Excessive, unexplained weight gain or loss
- Vital signs: blood pressure, temperature, pulse, respirations
- Insomnia
- Irritability
- Hoarseness or change in voice, frequent or prolonged sore throat
- Dizziness, falls

Integumentary (includes skin, hair, and nails)
- Recent rashes, nodules, or other skin changes
- Unusual hair loss or breakage
- Increased hair growth (hirsutism)
- Nail bed changes
- Itching (pruritus)

Musculoskeletal/Neurologic
- Joint pain, redness, warmth, swelling, stiffness, deformity

*Cluster of three to four or more, lasting longer than 1 month, is a red flag for immediate referral.

- Frequent or severe headaches
- Vision or hearing changes
- Vertigo
- Paresthesia (numbness, tingling, "pins and needles" sensation)
- Change in muscle tone
- Weakness; atrophy
- Abnormal deep tendon (or other) reflexes
- Problems with coordination or balance; falling
- Involuntary movements; tremors
- Radicular pain
- Seizures or loss of consciousness
- Memory loss
- Paralysis
- Mood swings; hallucinations

Rheumatologic
- Presence/location of joint swelling
- Muscle pain, weakness
- Skin rashes
- Reaction to sunlight
- Raynaud's phenomenon
- Nail bed changes

Cardiovascular
- Chest pain or sense of heaviness or discomfort
- Palpitations
- Limb pain during activity (claudication; cramps, limping)
- Discolored or painful feet; swelling of hands and feet
- Pulsating or throbbing pain anywhere, but especially in the back or abdomen
- Peripheral edema; nocturia
- Sudden weight gain; unable to fasten waist band or belt, unable to wear regular shoes
- Persistent cough
- Fatigue, dyspnea, orthopnea, syncope
- High or low blood pressure, unusual pulses
- Differences in blood pressure from side to side with position change (10 mm Hg or more; increase or decrease/diastolic or systolic; associated symptoms: dizziness, headache, nausea, vomiting, diaphoresis, heart palpitations, increased primary pain or symptoms)
- Positive findings on auscultation

Pulmonary
- Cough, hoarseness
- Sputum, hemoptysis
- Shortness of breath (dyspnea, orthopnea); altered breathing (e.g., wheezing, pursed-lip breathing)
- Night sweats
- Pleural pain
- Cyanosis, clubbing
- Positive findings on auscultation (e.g., friction rub, unexpected breath sounds)

Psychologic
- Sleep disturbance
- Stress levels
- Fatigue, psychomotor agitation
- Changes in personal habits, appetite
- Depression, confusion, anxiety
- Irritability, mood changes

Gastrointestinal
- Abdominal pain
- Indigestion; heartburn
- Difficulty in swallowing
- Nausea/vomiting; loss of appetite
- Diarrhea or constipation
- Change in stools; change in bowel habits
- Fecal incontinence
- Rectal bleeding; blood in stool; blood in vomit
- Skin rash followed by joint pain (Crohn's disease)

Hepatic/Biliary
- Change in taste/smell
- Anorexia
- Feeling of abdominal fullness, ascites
- Asterixis (muscle tremors)
- Change in urine color (dark, cola-colored)
- Light-colored stools
- Change in skin color (yellow, green)
- Skin changes (rash, itching, purpura, spider angiomas, palmar erythema)

Hematologic
- Skin color or nail bed changes
- Bleeding: nose, gums, easy bruising, melena

- Hemarthrosis, muscle hemorrhage, hematoma
- Fatigue, dyspnea, weakness
- Rapid pulse, palpitations
- Confusion, irritability
- Headache

Genitourinary

- Reduced stream, decreased output
- Burning or bleeding during urination; change in urine color
- Urinary incontinence, dribbling
- Impotence, pain with intercourse
- Hesitation, urgency
- Nocturia, frequency
- Dysuria (painful or difficult urination)
- Testicular pain or swelling
- Genital lesions
- Penile or vaginal discharge
- Impotence (males) or other sexual difficulty (males or females)
- Infertility (males or females)
- Flank pain

Gynecologic

- Irregular menses, amenorrhea, menopause
- Pain with menses or intercourse
- Vaginal discharge, vaginal itching
- Surgical procedures
- Pregnancy, birth, miscarriage, and abortion histories
- Spotting, bleeding—especially for the postmenopausal woman 12 months after last period (without hormone replacement therapy)

Endocrine

- Hair and nail changes
- Change in appetite, unexplained weight change
- Fruity breath odor
- Temperature intolerance, hot flashes, diaphoresis (unexplained perspiration)
- Heart palpitations, tachycardia
- Headaches
- Low urine output, absence of perspiration
- Cramps
- Edema, polyuria, polydipsia, polyphagia
- Unexplained weakness, fatigue, paresthesia

- Carpal/tarsal tunnel syndrome
- Periarthritis, adhesive capsulitis
- Joint or muscle pain (arthralgia, myalgia), trigger points
- Prolonged deep tendon reflexes
- Sleep disturbance

Cancer
- Constant, intense pain, especially bone pain at night
- Unexplained weight loss (10% of body weight in 10 to 14 days); most clients in pain are inactive and gain weight
- Loss of appetite
- Excessive fatigue
- Unusual lump(s), thickening, change in a lump or mole, sore that does not heal
- Other unusual skin lesions or rash
- Unusual or prolonged bleeding or discharge anywhere
- Change in bowel or bladder habits
- Chronic cough or hoarseness, change in voice
- Rapid onset of digital clubbing (10 to 14 days)
- (Proximal) muscle weakness, especially when accompanied by change in one or more deep tendon reflexes

Immunologic
- Skin or nail bed changes
- Fever or other constitutional symptoms (especially recurrent or cyclical symptoms)
- Lymph node changes (tenderness, enlargement)
- Anaphylactic reaction
- Symptoms of muscle or joint involvement (pain, swelling, stiffness, weakness)
- Sleep disturbance

OTHER TESTS AND MEASURES

Examples:

Emotional overlay (McGill Pain Questionnaire, Symptom Magnification, Waddell's nonorganic signs)

Special tests (e.g., Murphy's percussion, Obturator or Iliopsoas tests for abscess, abdominal aortic pulse, visceral palpation, auscultation of femoral bruits, Blumberg's sign, clinical breast exam, or other as appropriate)

Sample Upper Quarter Examination Sequence[4]

STANDING

Posture observation
Gait

SITTING*

General survey:
Skin, nails, hair, surface anatomy
Vital signs
Weight/height
Posture assessment (observe during the interview process)
Head, face, neck observation
Eyes
    Pupils
    Ptosis
    Visual gaze (strabismus)
Facial contour
    Eyes/mouth (CN VII)
    Cheeks (masseter muscle, CN V)
Intraoral
    Teeth (dentition and occlusion)
    Gingiva (gums)
    Tongue and other soft tissues
    Anterior neck (trachea and sternal notch)
Head, face, and neck palpation
    Glands (parotid, submandibular salivary, thyroid)
    Lymph nodes (preauricular and postauricular, suboccipital, tonsillar, submental, superficial and posterior cervical, supraclavicular)
    Trachea
    Carotid pulses
Head, face, and neck neurologic screening
    Follow-up interview questions
    Sense of smell (CN I)

*All positive neurologic findings in the sitting position should be retested in non-weight-bearing positions.
CN, Cranial nerve.

Visual acuity (CN II)
Diplopia (double vision) (CN III, IV, VI)
Sense of taste (CN VII, IX)
Difficulties with swallowing
Hearing loss
Numbness/paresthesia
Balance/gait difficulties
Mentation/orientation/behavioral abnormalities
Physical examination screening (optional)
    Smell (CN I)
    Visual acuity (CN II): Snellen eye chart
    Pupils: light reaction (CN II and III)
    Extraocular eye movements (CN III, IV, and/or VI)
    Sensory (CN V, and C2 and 3)
    Motor (CN V and VII, and C1 to C3)
    Motor cervical flexion (C1 to C3; CN XI: spinal accessory); extension (C1 to C8; CN XI: spinal accessory); lateral flexion (C2 to C4; CN XI); rotation
    Facial expression: eyes, mouth (CN VII)
    Hearing: air conduction (CN VIII)
    Hearing: bone conduction (CN VIII)
    Gag reflex (CN IX and X)
    Shoulder shrug (CN XI)
    Tongue motor response (CN XII)
Active range of motion (ROM) (with passive overpressure when appropriate)
    Mandibular depression (observe and palpate)
    Cervical spine
    Flexion
    Rotation (check vertebral artery signs)
    Lateral flexion
    Extension
    Cervical spine vertical compression/distraction
    Shoulder girdle/upper extremity
Observation
Palpation
    Lymph nodes (clavicular, axillary, and epitrochlear)
    Pulses (brachial, radial)
    Joint lines and soft tissues
Active ROM (with passive overpressure when appropriate)

Shoulder girdle
    Elevation, depression, protraction, retraction
Shoulder
    Hand behind head
    Hand behind back
    Horizontal abduction
Elbow (may do before shoulder's active ROM screening if history of significant elbow injury/pathology)
    Flexion
    Extension
    Pronation
    Supination
Wrist
    Flexion
    Extension
    Radial/ulnar deviation
Thumb
    Flexion/extension
    Opposition
Fingers
    Flexion/extension
Upper extremity neurologic screening
    Hoffman's reflex
    Cutaneous sensation (light touch, sharp/dull assessment) C4 to T6 dermatomes; see Myotome testing
        Scapular elevation (CN XI, spinal accessory)
        Shoulder abduction (C4 to C6, axillary)
        Elbow flexion (C5, C6; musculocutaneous)
        Elbow extension (C6 to C8, radial)
        Wrist extension (C6 to C8, radial and ulnar)
        Finger flexors (C7, C8; median)
        Thumb extension (C7, C8; radial)
        Finger abduction/adduction (C8, T1; ulnar)
    Deep tendon reflexes
        Biceps (C5, C6)
        Brachioradialis (C5, C6)
        Triceps (C6, C7)

Sample Lower Quarter Examination Sequence[4]

STANDING

- Postural observation
- General palpation
- Gait
- Inspection/palpation, including bony landmarks (ribs, iliac crests, posterior superior iliac spine [PSIS], greater trochanters, popliteal creases/fibular heads, malleoli, calcaneus, medial longitudinal arch, anterior superior iliac spine [ASIS], patella/tibial tuberosity, and forefoot including great toe)
- Standing squat (general clearing of the lumbar, pelvic, hip, knee, foot, and ankle regions)
- Vertical "quick" compression (heel bounce)
- Balance
    Bilateral stance
    Unilateral stance
- Active range of motion (AROM) trunk (with passive overpressures if symptoms not produced during the active movements); rotation to be done in sitting position
    Flexion
    Right and left lateral flexion
    Extension
- Neurologic screening; myotome and dermatome testing
- Heel raise (S1, S2) tibial nerve and superficial peroneal nerve
- Toe raise (L4, L5) deep peroneal nerve
- Sensation of posterior lower extremities (LEs) (S1, S2)

SITTING

- Posture (observe during the interview process)
- Active trunk rotation and overpressures
- Thoracic cage: upper and lower respiratory excursion
- Vertical trunk compression and decompression (spine in neutral position)
- Neurologic screening:
    Sensory
        Trunk: anterior (T7–T12; abdomen)
        LEs: L1–S1 (anterior, medial, lateral)

Myotome
> Trunk (multisegmental and peripheral nerves) flexion, extension, lateral flexion
>
> LEs
>
> Hip flexion: L1, L2, L3 (femoral nerve)
>
> Adduction: L1, L2, L3 (obturator nerve)
>
> Abduction: L4, L5, S1 (sup/inf gluteal nerve)
>
> Knee extension: L2, L3, L4 (femoral nerve)
>
> Knee flexion: L4, L5, S1, S2 (sciatic-tibial nerve)
>
> Dorsiflexion: L4, L5 (deep peroneal nerve)
>
> Extensor hallucis longus: L5–S1 (deep peroneal nerve)
>
> Eversion: L5–S1 (superficial peroneal nerve)
>
> NOTE: already have tested plantar flexors in standing position (S1 and S2, tibial nerve)

Deep tendon reflexes (DTR)
> Patellar tendon: (L2, L3, L4)
>
> Achilles tendon: (S1, S2)

SUPINE

- Posture (compare with standing position findings)
- General palpation (compare with standing position findings)
- Neck flexion dural tension testing
- Thorax/abdomen
  > Layer palpation of abdominal region
  >
  > Abdominal aorta (width and strength of pulse); auscultate if have concerns about the involvement of the aorta (see Chapter 9)
  >
  > Sensory T7–T12 anterior aspect
  >
  > Superficial abdominal reflex (T7–L1)
  >
  > Femoral triangle palpation
  >
  > Pulses: femoral artery auscultation for bruit if indicated
  >
  > Lymph nodes: inguinal nodes: vertical and horizontal chains
- Lower extremity palpation
- Pulses (popliteal artery, posterior tibial artery, dorsalis pedis artery)
- Sacroiliac (SI) gap, compression testing, and ilial shear testing
- Trunk AROM: double knee to chest
- AROM/Passive range of motion (PROM) lower extremities (LE) (add overpressures if symptoms not produced during AROM)

Knee flexion and extension
Hip flexion
Hip internal and external rotation
FABER (flexion, abduction, and external rotation)/FADIR (flexion, adduction, and internal rotation)

- Ankle dorsiflexion (knee flexed and extended; gastrocnemius versus soleus) and plantar flexion
    Ankle inversion and eversion
    Toe flexion and extension
- Straight leg raise
- Neurologic screening
- Babinski's test
- Repeat or include any or all myotome, sensory, and deep tendon reflex (DTR) tests that were positive in sitting or standing, or were not done previously

PRONE

- Postural observation (compared with other positions and with normal)
- Palpation of posterior lower quarter, as in standing
- AROM/PROM (add overpressures if symptoms not produced during AROM)
    Prone press-up (if standing trunk extension was symptomatic)
    Knee flexion
    Hip extension
- Neurologic screening
    Sensory testing: S1 to S2 (S2, S3, S4: anal region if patient reports any symptoms suggestive of cauda equina)
    Myotome testing: hip extension (L5, S1, S2: gluteal and tibial nerves)
    Femoral nerve tension test

Tests and Measures Used in the Physical Therapy Examination[1,38,54]

Test	Description	Issues Examined
Aerobic capacity	Ability to use the body's O_2 uptake and delivery system	• During functional activities • During standardized exercise testing • Signs and symptoms of cardiovascular system in response to increased oxygen demand during increased activity • Signs and symptoms of pulmonary system in response to increased oxygen demand during increased activity
Anthropometric characteristics	Body measurements and fat composition	• Body composition • Body dimensions • Edema
Arousal, attention, cognition	Degree of responsiveness and awareness	Motivation
Assistive/adaptive devices	Equipment to aid in performing tasks	• Equipment or devices used during functional activities • Components, alignment, fit, and ability to care for devices or equipment • Effectiveness of devices or equipment in correcting impairments, limitations, or disabilities • Safety during use of equipment or devices
Circulation	Analysis of blood and lymph movement to determine adequacy of cardiovascular pump, oxygen delivery, and lymphatic drainage	• Cardiovascular signs • Physiological responses to position changes
Cranial/peripheral nerve integrity	Assessment of sensory and motor functions of cranial and peripheral nerves	• Motor distribution and integrity • Sensory distribution and integrity
Environmental barriers	Analysis of physical restrictions to functioning in the environment	Physical space and environment

Continued

Test	Description	Issues Examined
Ergonomics/body mechanics	Analyses of work tasks and postural adjustment to perform tasks	• Coordination and dexterity during functional activities • Functional and physical performance during work tasks • Safety in work environment • Specific work conditions/activities • Tools, equipment, and workstation design used during job activities • Body mechanics during home and work activities
Gait and balance	Analyses of walking, moving from place to place, and equilibrium	• Static and dynamic balance with or without the use of assistive devices or prosthetics • Balance during functional activities with or without the use of assistive devices or prosthetics • Gait during functional activities with or without the use of assistive devices or prosthetics • Safety during gait and balance activities
Integumentary integrity	Health of the skin	• Activities and positioning that produce or relieve trauma to the skin • Equipment, devices, or prosthesis that may produce trauma to the skin • Current skin characteristics and conditions • Activities or positioning that may aggravate the wound or scar • Presence of signs of infection • Wound/scar characteristics
Joint integrity and mobility	Assessment of joint structure and impact on passive movement	Joint play including accessory movements
Motor function	Control of voluntary movement	• Dexterity, coordination, and agility • Hand function
Muscle performance	Analysis of muscle strength, power, and endurance	• Strength, power, and endurance • Strength, power, and endurance during functional activities • Muscle tension

Test	Description	Issues Examined
Neuromotor development and sensory integration	Evolution of movement skills and integration of information from the environment	• Development of motor skills • Speech production, phonation, and oral motor function • Sensorimotor integration: postural, equilibrium, etc.
Orthotic, protective, and supportive devices	Determination of need for fit of devices to support weak joints	• Components, alignment, and fit of devices • Use during functional activities • Effectiveness of devices in correcting limitations and disabilities • Safety during use of devices
Pain	Analysis of intensity, quality, and frequency of pain	• Location and description of pain • Intensity ratings of pain
Posture	Analysis of body alignment and positioning	• Postural alignment and positioning, static and dynamic • Alignment of specific body parts
Prosthetic requirements	Selection, fit, and use of prostheses	• Components, alignment, fit, and ability to care for prosthesis • Use of prosthesis during functional activities • Effectiveness of prosthesis at correcting limitations, impairments, and disabilities • Residual limb edema, strength, ROM, and skin integrity • Safety during use of prosthesis
Reflex integrity	Assessment of developmental, normal, and pathological reflexes	• Deep, postural, primitive, and superficial reflexes • Resistance and reactions
ROM	Amount of movement at a joint	• Functional ROM • Active and passive joint movement • Muscle length and flexibility, soft tissue extensibility
Self-care and home management	Analysis of activities necessary for independent living at home	• Ability to access home • Ability to perform self-care and home management activities • Safety in home and self-care management

Continued

continued from p. 65

Test	Description	Issues Examined
Sensory integrity	Assessment of peripheral and central sensory processing, awareness of movement, and position	• Superficial sensation • Deep sensation • Combined/cortical sensation
Ventilation and respiration/gas exchange	Assessment of movement of air into and out of the lungs, exchange of gases, and transport of blood to perform activities of daily living and exercises	Pulmonary signs of respiration, ventilatory functions, and symptoms
Work/community/leisure integration	Analyses to determine whether the patient/client can assume a role in community or work	• Ability to return to work, community, and leisure activities • Ability to access work site, community, and leisure activities • Safety in work, community, and leisure activities

ROM, Range of motion.
Format and terminology consistent with *Guide to Physical Therapist Practice*

Pediatric Physical Therapy Assessments[51,57,66]

Assessment	Age Range	Measures
Alberta Infant Motor Scale (AIMS)	Birth–18 mos	Identifies motor delays and measures changes in motor performance over time Prone, supine, sit, and stand
Batelle Developmental Inventory	Birth–8 yrs	Identifies developmental level and monitors changes over time
Bayley Scales of Infant Development, 2nd ed. (BSID-II)	1–42 mos	Identifies developmental delay in gross motor, fine motor, and cognitive domains; monitors progress over time
Berg Balance Scale	5 yrs and older	Performance-based measure of balance during specific movement tasks
Bruininks-Oseretsky Test of Motor Proficiency (BOTMP)	4.5–14.5 yrs	Gross and fine motor, bilateral coordination Tests bilateral coordination and balance; monitor change over longer periods of time for child with mild disabilities
Canadian Occupational Performance Measure (COPM)	Any age	Identifies changes in parent or child's self-perception of performance over time
Child Health Questionnaire	2 mos–15 yrs	Measures quality of life from patient's or parents' perspective

Assessment	Age Range	Measures
Denver (DDDST II)	1 wk–6.5 yrs	Motor, cognitive, language, social, and adaptive Quick and easy to learn
Early Intervention Developmental Profile	Birth–3 yrs	Developmental screening
Energy Expenditure Index (EEI)	3 yrs and older	Measures endurance level for activity; monitors changes over time
Functional Independence Measure for Children (WeeFIM)	6 mos–7 yrs	Measures changes in mobility and activities of daily living (ADL) skills. Used for program evaluation and rehabilitation outcomes assessment
Functional Reach Test (FRT)	4 yrs and older	Measures anticipatory standing balance during reach
Gross Motor Function Measure (GMFM)	5 mos–16 yrs	Motor function in: 1. Lying and rolling 2. Sitting 3. Crawling and kneeling 4. Standing 5. Walking, running, and jumping Used to document progress in children with cerebral palsy (CP)
Hawaii Early Learning Profile	Birth–6 yrs	1. Cognition 2. Gross motor 3. Fine motor 4. Social 5. Self-help
Home Observation Measurement of the Environment (HOME)	Birth–10 yrs	Quantity and quality of stimulation in the home environment
Modified Ashworth Scale (MAS)	4 yrs and older	Qualitative measurement of spasticity via resistance to passive joint movement
Modified Tardieu Scale	4 yrs and older	Qualitative measurement of spasticity via resistance to passive joint movement
Movement Assessment of Infants (MAI)	Birth–12 mos	Identifies motor abilities or dysfunction
Peabody Developmental Motor Scales (PDMS-2)	Birth–5 yrs	Identifies gross and fine motor delays; used to monitor progress
Pediatric Clinical Test of Sensory Integration for Balance (P-CTSIB)	4–10 yrs	Measures sensory system contributions to standing balance and postural control
Pediatric Evaluation of Disability Inventory (PEDI)	6 mos–7.5 yrs	Self-care Ability Social function
Revised Gesell and Amatruda Developmental and Neurologic Examination	4 wks–36 mos	Identify minor deviations in development of gross motor, fine motor, language, and personal/social adaptive domains

Continued

continued from p. 67

Assessment	Age Range	Measures
School Function Assessment (SFA)	Kindergarten–6th grade	Participation Task support Activity performance Physical tasks Cognitive and behavioral tasks
Sensory Integration and Praxis Test	4–9 yrs	Measures sensory systems' contribution to balance and motor coordination
Sensory Profile	3–10 yrs	Determines which sensory processes contribute to child's performance with ADLs
6-Minute Walk Test	5 yrs and older	Measures walking endurance; monitors progress over time
Test of Gross Motor Development-2nd ed. (TGMD-2)	3–10 yrs	Locomotor and object control skills
Test of Infant Motor Performance (TIMP)	Infants 32 wks post-conception to 4 mos postterm	Provides early identification of motor delay; assesses postural control for early skills acquisition
Test of Sensory Function in Infants	4–18 mos	Identifies sensory processing dysfunction and those at risk for developmental delay or learning problems
Timed Up and Go (TUG)	4 yrs and older	Performance-based measure of anticipatory standing balance, gait and motor function
Toddler and Infant Motor Evaluation (TIME)	4 mos–3.5 yrs	Identifies children with mild-to-severe motor problems. Measures sensory development. Monitors progress over time.

CP, Cerebral palsy.

Sample List of Examination Tools[66]

Balance and Postural Control Tests

Clinical Scale of Contraversive Pushing
Clinical Test of Sensory Interaction on Balance (CTSIB)
Computerized Dynamic Posturography
Dix-Hallpike Test
Dynamic Visual Acuity and Gaze Stabilization Tests
Fukuda Stepping Test
Functional Reach Lateral
Functional Reach Test
Head-Shake SOT

Lateropulsion Test
Limits of Stability (LOS) Test on NeuroCom System
Modified Functional Reach Test
Multidirectional Reach Test
Nudge/Push Test
One Leg Stand Test
Postural Stress Test
Postural Sway Tests
Repetitive Reach Test
Romberg Test
Sensory Organization Test (SOT)
Sharpened Romberg Test

Functional Tests of Balance and Mobility

Berg Balance Scale (BBS)
Continuous-Scale Physical Functional Performance (CS-PFP)
Dynamic Gait Index (DGI)
Fast Evaluation of Mobility, Balance, and Fear (FEMBAF)
Four Square Step Test (FSST)
Gait and Balance Scale (GABS)
L-Test
Physical Performance and Mobility Examination (PPME)
Physical Performance Test (PPT)
Tandem Gait Test
Tinetti Performance-Oriented Mobility Assessment (POMA)
Timed Up and Go Test (TUG and mTUG)
Timed Movement Battery
Time Sit to Stand Test

Gait Tests

Automated Up-Timer
Clinical Gait Assessments
Functional Ambulation Profile
Functional Gait Assessment (FGA)
GAITRite System
Modified Gait Abnormality Rating Scale (GARS-M)
Observational Gait Analysis (Rancho)
5-Meter Walk Test
400-Meter Walk Test

2-Minute Walk Test
6-Minute Walk Test
12-Minute Walk Test

Falls Efficacy and Falls Prediction Scales

Activities-Specific Balance Confidence (ABC) Scale
Falls Efficacy Scale (FES)
Multiple Tasks Test (MTT)
Survey of Activities and Fear of Falling in the Elderly (SAFE)

Activities of Daily Living Scales

Barthel Index
Bristol Activities of Daily Living Scale
Katz Index of Activities of Daily Living
Kenny Self-Care Evaluation
Klein-Bell Activities of Daily Living Scale
Melville-Nelson Self-Care Assessment
PULSES Profile
Structured Assessment of Independent Living Skills (SAILS)
The Safety Assessment of Function and the Environment for Rehabilitation (SAFER)

Nonequilibrium Coordination Tests

Coordination Tests

Strength Tests

Grip Strength Dynamometry
Isokinetic Testing
Manual Muscle Test (MMT)

Range of Motion Tests

Objective Measurements of Joint Range of Motion

Spasticity and Tone Tests

Ashworth Scale
Modified Ashworth Scale
Tardieu Scale
Tone Assessment Scale

Cognitive Function, Dementia, Alzheimer's Tests

Abbreviated Mental Test (AMT)
Clock Drawing Test for Dementia Severity in Alzheimer's
Discomfort Assessment for Alzheimer's
Draw a Man Test (neglect)
Mental Status Questionnaire (MSQ)
Mini-Mental State Examination (MMSE)
Modified Mini-Mental State Examination (3MS)
Multidimensional Observation Scale for Elderly Subjects (MOSES)
Orientation Log (O-LOG)
Rancho Los Amigos Levels of Cognitive Functioning Assessment Scale (LOCFAS)
Recognition Memory Test (RMT)
Short Portable Mental Status Questionnaire (SPMSQ)
Supervision Rating Scale (SRS)
Wisconsin Card Sorting Test (WCST-64)

Depression Scales

Aphasic Depression Scale
Beck Depression Inventory
Geriatric Depression Scale
Hamilton Rating Scale for Depression
Montgomery-Asberg Depression Scale
Zung Depression Scale

Coma Scales

Coma/Near Coma (CNC) Scale
Coma Recovery Scale (CRS)
Glasgow Coma Scale (GCS)
Glasgow Epilepsy Outcome Scale (GEOS)
Glasgow Outcome Scale (GOS)
Western Neuro Sensory Stimulation Profile (WNSSP)

Amnesia Scales

Children's Orientation and Amnesia Test (COAT)
Galveston Orientation and Amnesia Test (GOAT)
Post Traumatic Amnesia Scale (PTA)
Wolinsky Amnesia Information Test (WAIT)

Stroke Tools

American Heart Association Stroke Outcome Classification Scale
Arm Motor Ability Test (AMAT)
Box and Block Test
Chedoke Arm and Hand Inventory
Chedoke-McMaster Stroke Assessment
Frenchay Activities Index (FAI)
Fugl-Meyer
Lateropulsion Scale for Stroke
LIDO Active System: Resistance to Passive Shoulder ER
Lower Extremity Motor Coordination Test (LEMOCO)
Modified Berg Balance Scale for Stroke (BBS-3P)
Modified Motor Assessment Scale (MMAS)
Motor Assessment Scale (MAS)
Motor Status Score (MSS)
National Institutes of Health Stroke Scale (NIHSS)
Postural Assessment in Stroke Scale (PASS)
Rankin Scale
Reaching Performance Scale
Rivermead Mobility Index (RMI)
Scandinavian Stroke Supervision Scale
Sodring Motor Evaluation of Stroke (SMES)
Stroke-Adapted 30-Item Sickness Impact Profile (SA-SIP 30)
Stroke Rehabilitation Assessment of Movement (STREAM)
Trunk Control Test (TCT)
Trunk Impairment Scale (TIS)
Unified Neurological Stroke Scale (UFNSS)
Upright Motor Control Test
Wolf Motor Function Test

Parkinson and Huntington Disease Tools

Dyskinesia Rating Scales
Parkinson Disease Questionnaire (PDQ-39)
Unified Huntington Disease Rating Scale (UHDRS)
Unified Parkinson Disease Rating Scale (UPDRS)

Multiple Sclerosis Tools

Cambridge Multiple Sclerosis Basic Score (CAMBS)
Disease Steps

EQUI-SCALE
Fahn's Tremor Rating Scale (FTRS)
Functional Assessment of Multiple Sclerosis (FAMS)
Functional Limitations Profile (FLP)
Kurtzke Extended Disability Status Scale (EDDS)
Multiple Sclerosis Functional Composite Measure (MSFC)
Multiple Sclerosis Symptom Inventory (MSSI)
Scripps Neurological Rating Scale (SNRS)
The Multiple Sclerosis Impairment Scale (MSIS)

Spinal Cord Injury Tools

American Spinal Injury Association (ASIA) Functional Classification of Spinal Cord Injury
Capabilities of Upper Extremity (CUE) Test
FIM for SCI with 5 Additional Mobility and Locomotor items (5-AML)
Quadriplegia Index of Function (QIF)
Self-Care Assessment Tool (SCAT)
Walking Index for Spinal Cord Injury (WISCI)

Select Orthopedic Tools

Fibromyalgia Tools
Functional Rating Index (FRI)
Low Back Pain Questionnaires and Functional Measures
Physical Function Health Status (FHS)
Shoulder Questionnaires
Total Joint Replacement Tests
Western Ontario Shoulder Instability Index (WOSI)

Pain Assessment Tools

Back Pain Functional Scale (BPFS)
Back Performance Scale
Brief Pain Inventory (BPI)
Dartmouth Pain Questionnaire
Functional Pain Scale (FPS)
General Function Score
Million Visual Analog Scale (VAS)
Neck Pain and Disability Scale

Oswestry Low Back Pain Disability Questionnaire
Pain Disability Index (PDI)
Pain-O-Meter
Patient-Specific Functional Scale
Quebec Back Pain Disability Questionnaire
Roland-Morris Back Pain Disability Questionnaire
Shoulder Pain and Disability Index (SPADI)
Wheelchair Users Subjective Pain Index (WUSPI)

Health Status Tools: Disability, Handicap

Arthritis Impact Scale
Disability Rating Scale (DRS)
Dizziness Handicap Inventory (DHI)
Fibromyalgia Health Assessment Questionnaire (FHAQ)
Fibromyalgia Impact Questionnaire
Frail Elderly Functional Assessment Questionnaire (FEFA)
Functional Assessment Measure (FIM+FAM)
Functional Independence Measure (FIM)
Functional Status Examination for TBI (FSE)
Hospital Admission Risk Profile (HARP)
McMaster University Osteoarthritis Index
Musculoskeletal Function Assessment Questionnaire
Nottingham Health Profile
OASIS
Pain Disability Questionnaire (PDQ)
Patient Health Questionnaire-9 for TBI (PHQ-9)
Pediatric Quality of Life Instrument (Peds QL)
Physical Disability Index (PDI)
Short-Form 36 Health Survey Questionnaire (SF-36)
Sickness Impact Profile (SIP & SIP 68)
Subjective Index and Physical and Social Outcome (SIPSO) (for
    Stroke)
Functional Independence Measure for Children (WeeFIM)
Western Ontario Osteoarthritis Index

Pediatric Tools

Alberta Infant Motor Scale
Assessment Evaluation and Programming System for Infants and
    Children

Ages and Stages Questionnaire

Batelle Developmental Inventory

Bayley Infant Neurodevelopmental Screener

Bayley Scales of Infant Development

Bruininks-Oseretsky Test of Motor Proficiency (BOTMP)

Canadian Occupational Performance Measure

Child Health Questionnaire (CHQ)

Child Health Assessment Questionnaire (CHAQ)

Children's Orientation and Amnesia Scale (COAT)

Clinical Observation of Motor and Postural Skills Test (COMPS)

The Carolina Curriculum for Infants and Toddlers with Special Needs

The Carolina Curriculum for Preschoolers with Special Needs

DENVER II

Erhardt Developmental Prehension Assessment (EDPA)

Functional Independence Measure for Children (WeeFIM)

Gillette Functional Assessment Questionnaire

Gross Motor Function Measure (GMFM)

Infant Motor Screen (IMS)

Infant Neurological International Battery (INFANIB)

Milani-Comparetti Motor Development Screening Test

Movement Assessment of Infants (MAI)

Neurological Assessment of the Preterm and Full-Term New Born Infant (NAPFI)

Neurobehavioral Assessment of Preterm Infant (NAPI)

Neonatal Behavioral Assessment Scale (NBAS)

Neonatal Neurobehavioral Examination (NNE)

Neonatal Oral Motor Assessment Scale (NOMAS)

Peabody Developmental Motor Scales

Pediatric Clinical Test of Sensory Interaction on Balance (P-CTSIB)

Pediatric Evaluation of Disability Inventory (PEDI)

Pediatric Quality of Life Instrument (Peds QL)

Infant/Toddler Sensory Profile

School Function Assessment (SFA)

Sensory Integration and Praxis Test

Test of Infant Motor Performance (TIMP)

Toddler and Infant Motor Evaluation (TIME)

Example of an Assessment form[39]

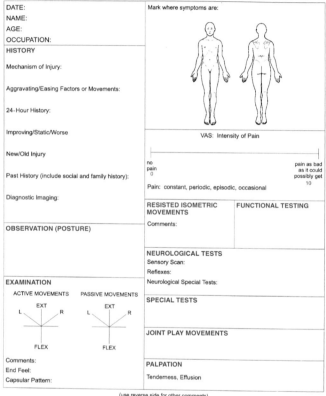

DATE:
NAME:
AGE:
OCCUPATION:

HISTORY

Mechanism of Injury:

Aggravating/Easing Factors or Movements:

24-Hour History:

Improving/Static/Worse

New/Old Injury

Past History (include social and family history):

Diagnostic Imaging:

OBSERVATION (POSTURE)

EXAMINATION

ACTIVE MOVEMENTS   PASSIVE MOVEMENTS

EXT   EXT
L   R   L   R

FLEX   FLEX

Comments:
End Feel:
Capsular Pattern:

Mark where symptoms are:

VAS: Intensity of Pain

no
pain   pain as bad
0   as it could
                                                      possibly get
                                                      10
Pain: constant, periodic, episodic, occasional

RESISTED ISOMETRIC   **FUNCTIONAL TESTING**
MOVEMENTS

Comments:

NEUROLOGICAL TESTS
Sensory Scan:
Reflexes:
Neurological Special Tests:

SPECIAL TESTS

JOINT PLAY MOVEMENTS

PALPATION

Tenderness, Effusion

(use reverse side for other comments)

Posture Assessment

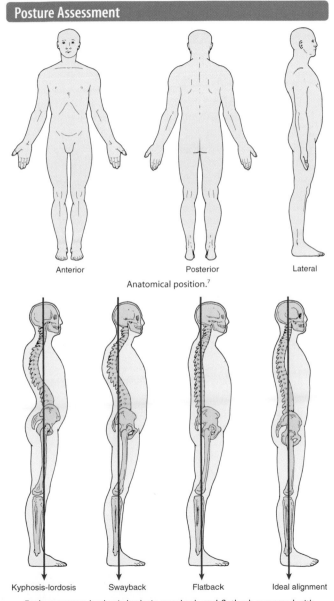

Anterior   Posterior   Lateral

Anatomical position.[7]

Kyphosis-lordosis   Swayback   Flatback   Ideal alignment

Faulty postures: kyphosis-lordosis, swayback, and flatback compared with ideal alignment.[7]

Joint Range of Motion and Muscle-Length Testing

PROCEDURES FOR MEASURING JOINT RANGE OF MOTION AND MUSCLE LENGTH[59]

1. Determine the type of measurement to be performed (AROM or PROM).
2. Explain the purpose of the procedure to the patient.
3. Position the patient in the preferred patient position for the measurement.
4. Stabilize the proximal joint segment.
5. Instruct the patient in the specific motion that will be measured while moving the patient's distant joint segment passively through the ROM. Determine the patient's end-feel at the end of the PROM.
6. Return the patient's distal joint segment to the starting position.
7. Palpate bony landmarks for measurement-device alignment.
8. Align the measurement device with the appropriate bony landmarks.
9. Read the scale of the measurement device and note the reading.
10. Have the patient move actively, or move the patient passively, through the available ROM.
11. Repalpate the bony landmarks and readjust the alignment of the measurement device as necessary.
12. Read the scale of the measurement device and note the reading.
13. Record the patient's ROM. The record should include, at a minimum:
    a. Patient's name and identifying information
    b. Date measurement was taken
    c. Identification of person taking measurement
    d. Type of motion measured (AROM or PROM) and device used
    e. Any alteration from preferred patient position
    f. Readings taken from measurement device at beginning and end of ROM

SUGGESTED VALUES FOR NORMAL RANG OF MOTION FOR JOINTS OF THE UPPER AND LOWER EXTREMITY IN ADULTS BASED ON ANALYSIS OF EXISTING DATA[59]

Joint	ROM
UPPER EXTREMITY	
Shoulder	
FLEXION	0°–165°
EXTENSION	0°–60°
ABDUCTION	0°–165°
MEDIAL ROTATION	0°–70°
LATERAL ROTATION	0°–90°
Elbow	
FLEXION	0°–140°
EXTENSION	0°
Forearm	
PRONATION	0°–80°
SUPINATION	0°–80°
Wrist	
FLEXION	0°–80°
EXTENSION	0°–70°
ABDUCTION (RADIAL DEVIATION)	0°–20°
ADDUCTION (ULNAR DEVIATION)	0°–30°
1st Carpometacarpal Joint	
FLEXION	0°–15°
EXTENSION	0°–20°
ABDUCTION	0°–70°
Metacarpophalangeal Joints	
FLEXION	
Thumb	0°–50°
Fingers	0°–90°
EXTENSION	
Thumb	0°
Fingers	0°–20°
Interphalangeal Joints	
FLEXION	
IP joint (thumb)	0°–65°
PIP joint (fingers)	0°–100°
DIP joint (fingers)	0°–70°
EXTENSION	
IP joint (thumb)	0°–10° to 20°
PIP joint (fingers)	0°
DIP joints (fingers)	0°

Continued

Joint	ROM
LOWER EXTREMITY	
Hip	
FLEXION	0°–120°
EXTENSION	0°–20°
ABDUCTION	0°–40° to 45°
ADDUCTION	0°–25° to 30°
MEDIAL ROTATION	0°–35° to 40°
LATERAL ROTATION	0°–35° to 40°
Knee	
FLEXION	0°–140° to 145°
EXTENSION	0°
Ankle/Foot	
DORSIFLEXION*	0°–15° to 20°
PLANTAR FLEXION†	0°–40° to 50°
INVERSION†	0°–30° to 35°
EVERSION*	0°–20°
1st Metatarsophalangeal (MTP) Joint	
FLEXION	0°–20°
EXTENSION	0°–80°

IP, Interphalangeal; *PIP*, proximal interphalangeal; *DIP*, distal interphalangeal.
*Component of pronation. (ROM values apply to foot, not to isolated subtalar joint, motion.)
†Component of supination. (ROM values apply to foot, not to isolated subtalar joint, motion.)

TRADITIONALLY QUOTED VALUES FOR NORMAL RANGE OF MOTION FOR JOINTS OF THE UPPER AND LOWER EXTREMITY IN ADULTS[59]

Joint	ROM Values	
UPPER EXTREMITY		
	AAOS, 1965	AMA, 1993
Shoulder		
FLEXION	0–180°	0–180°
EXTENSION	0–60°	0–50°
ABDUCTION	0–180°	0–180°
MEDICAL ROTATION	0–70°	0–90°
Elbow		
FLEXION	0–150°	0–140°
EXTENSION	0°	0°
Forearm		
PRONATION	0–80°	0–80°
SUPINATION	0–80°	0–80°

Joint	ROM Values	
Wrist		
FLEXION	0–80°	0–80°
EXTENSION	0–70°	0–60°
ABDUCTION (RADIAL DEVIATION)	0–20°	0–20°
ADDUCTION (ULNAR DEVIATION)	0–30°	0–30°
1St Carpometacarpal Joint		
FLEXION	0–15°	
EXTENSION	0–20°	0–50°
ABDUCTION	0–70°	
Metacarpophalangeal Joints		
FLEXION		
Thumb	0–50°	0–60°
Fingers	0–90°	0–90°
EXTENSION		
Thumb	0°	0°
Fingers	0–45°	0–45°
Interphalangeal Joints		
FLEXION		
IP joint (thumb)	0–80°	0–80°
PIP joint (fingers)	0–100°	0–100°
DIP joint (fingers)	0–90°	0–70°
EXTENSION		
IP joint (thumb)	0–20°	0–10°
PIP joints (fingers)	0°	0°
DIP joint (fingers)	0°	0°
LOWER EXTREMITY		
	AAOS, 1965	AMA, 1984
Hip		
FLEXION	0°–120°	0°–100°
EXTENSION	0°–30°	0°–30°
ABDUCTION	0°–45°	0°–40°
ADDUCTION	0°–30°	0°–20°
MEDIAL ROTATION	0°–45°	0°–50°
LATERAL ROTATION	0°–45°	0°–40°
Knee		
FLEXION	0°–135°	0°–150°
EXTENSION	0°–10°	0°
Ankle/Foot		
DORSIFLEXION[r]	0°–20°	0°–20°
PLANTAR FLEXION[§]	0°–50°	0°–40°
INVERSION[§]	0°–35°	0°–30°
EVERSION[§]	0°–15°	0°–20°

Continued

continued from p. 81

Joint	ROM Values	
1st Metatarsophalangeal (MTP) Joint		
FLEXION	0°–45°	0°–30°
EXTENSION	0°–70°	0°–50°

IP, Interphalangeal; *PIP*, proximal interphalangeal; *DIP*, distal interphalangeal; *AAOS*, American Academy of Orthopaedic Surgeons; *AMA*, American Medical Association.
‡Component of pronation.
§Component of supination.
(From Reese, NB: *Joint Range of Motion and Muscle Length Testing.* W.B. Saunders, Philadelphia, 2002.)

TRADITIONALLY QUOTED VALUES FOR NORMAL RANGE OF MOTION OF THE THORACIC AND LUMBAR SPINE IN ADULTS[59]

Motion	Schober*	Goniometer†	Inclinometer‡
Flexion	3–5 cm	90°	60°
Extension	—	30°	25°
Lateral flexion	—	30°	25°
Rotation	—	—	30°

*From Rothschild BM: *Rheumatology: a primary care approach.* Brooklyn, NY, Yorke Medical Books, 1982.
†Measurement of thoracolumbar spine norms provided by the American Medical Association.[2]
‡Measurement of rotation is for thoracic spine; all other measures are lumbar spine. Norms provided by the American Medical Association.[5]

SUGGESTED VALUES FOR NORMAL RANGE OF MOTION OF THE THORACIC AND LUMBAR SPINE IN ADULTS[59]

Motion	Modified Schober	Goniometer	Inclinometer
Flexion	6–7 cm	90°	60°
Extension	—	30°	30°
Lateral flexion	—	35°	30°
Rotation	—	—	6°

SUGGESTED VALUES FOR NORMAL RANGE OF MOTION OF CERVICAL SPINE IN ADULTS[59]

Motion	Tape Measure*	Gonlometer[†]	Nclinometer[‡]	Crom[§]
Flexion	1–4 cm	45°	50°	50°
Extension	20 cm	45°	60°	75°
Lateral flexion	15 cm	45°	45°	45°
Rotation	10 cm	—	80°	70°

CROM, Cervical range of motion device.

Note: The American Academy of Orthopedic Surgeons[5] does not provide normative data using a tape measure, inclinometer, or CROM.

*Cervical spine norms derived from data by Balogun et al.[4] and Hsieh and Yeung.[6]

†Cervical spine norms provided by the American Medical Association.[2]

‡Cervical spine norms provided by the American Medical Association.[3]

§Cervical spine norms derived from means of male and female data from ages 20–40 years according to study by Youdas et al.[7]

ADDITIONAL ROM REFERENCES

1. American Academy of Orthopaedic Surgeons: *Joint motion: method of measuring and recording*, Chicago, 1965, American Academy of Orthopaedic Surgeons.

2. American Medical Association: *Guides to the evaluation of permanent impairment*, 2nd ed, Chicago, 1984.

3. American Medical Association: *Guides to the evaluation of permanent impairment*, 4th ed, Chicago, 1993.

4. Balogun JA, Abereoje OK, Olaogun MO et al: Inter- and intratester reliability of measuring neck motions with tape measure and Myrin gravity-reference goniometer, *J Orthop Sports Phys Ther* 10:248–253, 1989.

5. Greene WB, Heckman JD: *The clinical measurement of joint motion*, Rosemont, Ill.

6. Hsieh C, Yeung B: Active neck motion measurements with a tape measure, *J Orthop Sports Phys Ther* 8:88–92, 1986.

7. Youdas JW, Garrett TR, Suman VJ et al: Normal range of motion of the cervical spine: An initial goniometric study, *Phys Ther* 72:770–780, 1992.

MUSCLE TEST GRADES[60]

Number (and Letter) Grade	Word Grade	Definition
0	Zero	No evidence of contraction by vision or palpation
1 (Tr)	Trace	Slight contraction; no motion
2– (P–)	Poor minus	Movement through partial test range in gravity-eliminated position
2 (P)	Poor	Movement through complete test range in gravity-eliminated position
2+ (P+)	Poor plus	Movement through complete test range in gravity-eliminated position and through up to one half of test range against gravity
3– (F–)	Fair minus	Movement through complete test range in gravity-eliminated position and through more than one half of test range against gravity
3 (F)	Fair	Movement through complete test range against gravity
3+ (F+)	Fair plus	Movement through complete test range against gravity and able to hold against minimum resistance
4 (G)	Good	Movement through complete test range against gravity and able to hold against moderate resistance
5 (N)	Normal	Movement through complete test range against gravity and able to hold against maximum resistance

Determinants of Gait[19]

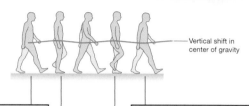

Vertical shift in center of gravity

Pelvic rotation in transverse plane minimizes drop in center of gravity by effectively lengthening the limbs

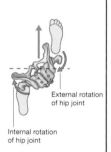

External rotation of hip joint

Internal rotation of hip joint

Movement of knees towards midline (adduction of hip) minimizes lateral shift in center of gravity

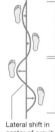

With adduction of hip (knees move toward midline)

No adduction of hip (knees do not move toward midline)

Lateral shift in center of gravity

Knee flexion on full stance. Limb minimizes rise in center of gravity by effectively shortening the limb

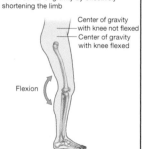

Center of gravity with knee not flexed
Center of gravity with knee flexed

Flexion

Pelvic tilt (drop) on swing side minimizes rise in center of gravity

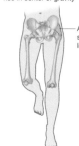

Abduction on stance side controls and limits the drop

Example of a Pain Assessment Tool[30]

TRANSLATIONS OF WONG-BAKER FACES PAIN RATING SCALE

	0-5 coding	0	1	2	3	4	5
	0-10 coding	0	2	4	6	8	10
ENGLISH		No hurt	Hurts little bit	Hurts little more	Hurts even more	Hurts whole lot	Hurts worst
SPANISH		No duele	Duele un poco	Duele un poco más	Duele mucho	Duele mucho más	Duele el máximo
FRENCH		Pas mal	Un petit peu mal	Un peu plus mal	Encore plus mal	Très mal	Très très mal
ITALIAN		Non fa male	Fa male un poco	Fa male un po di piu	Fa male ancora di piu	Fa molto male	Fa maggiormente male
PORTUGUESE		Não doi	Doi um pouco	Doi um pouco mais	Doi muito	Doi muito mais	Doi o máximo
BOSNIAN		Ne boli	Boli samo malo	Boli malo više	Boli još više	Boli puno	Boli najviše
VIETNAMESE		Không dau	Hôi dau	Dau hôn chut	Dau nhiêu hôn	Dau thât nhiêu	Dau qua dô
CHINESE[†]		無痛	微痛	較痛	更痛	很痛	痛刺痛
GREEK		Δεν πονάι	Πονάι λίγο	Πονάι πιο Πολύ	Πονάι Πιο Πολύ	Πονάι πιο Πολύ	Πονάι Παρα Πολύ
ROMANIAN		Nu doare	Doare puțin	Doare un pic mai mult	Doare și mai mult	Doare foarte tare	Doare cel mai mult

Three Standard Spasticity Scales: Ashworth, Modified Ashworth, and Spasm Frequency[62]

Ashworth Scale

GRADE	DESCRIPTION
1	No increased tone
2	Slight increase in tone, giving a catch when the affected parts are moved in flexion or extension
3	More marked increased in tone but affected part is easily flexed
4	Considerable increase in tone, passive movement is difficult
5	Affected part is rigid in extension

Modified Ashworth Scale

GRADE	DESCRIPTION
0	No increased muscle tone
1	Slight increase in muscle tone, manifested by a catch and release, or by minimal resistance at end ROM when affected part is moved in flexion or extension
1+	Slight increase in muscle tone, manifested by a catch, followed by minimal resistance throughout the remainder (<50%) of ROM
2	More marked increase in muscle tone through most of ROM, but affected part is easily moved
3	Considerable increase in muscle tone, passive movement difficult
4	Affected part is rigid in flexion or extension

Spasm Frequency Score

GRADE	DESCRIPTION
0	No spasms
1	Mild spasm induced by stimulation
2	Infrequent full spasm occurring less than once per hour
3	Spasms occurring more than once per hour
4	Ten or more spasms per hour, or continuous contraction

Data from Ashworth B: Preliminary trial of carisoprodol in multiple sclerosis, *Practioner* 192:540–542, 1964; Bohannon RW, Smith MB: Interrator reliability on modified Ashworth scale of muscle spasticity, *Phys Ther* 67:206–207, 1987; Penn RD, Savoy SM, Corcos DC et al: Intrathecal baclofen for severe spinal spasticity, *N Engl J Med* 320:1517–1521, 1989.

Key Muscle Groups[62]

TEN MUSCLE GROUPS THAT ARE TESTED AS PART OF THE STANDARDIZED SPINAL CORD EXAMINATION

Root Level	Muscle Group
C5	Elbow flexors
C6	Wrist flexors
C7	Elbow extensors
C8	Long finger flexors
T1	Small finger abductors
L2	Hip flexors
L3	Knee flexors
L4	Ankle dorsiflexors
L5	Long toe extensor
S1	Ankle plantar flexors

Tests

Shoulder

ADSON'S TEST[39]

With the patient sitting, the clinician locates patient's radial pulse with elbow extended. The patient rotates his or her head toward test shoulder and extends head/neck. The therapist then externally rotates and extends the patient's shoulder as the patient takes a deep breath and holds it.

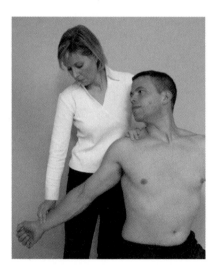

Positive sign: Reproduction of pain and paresthesia in tested upper extremity with diminished or absent pulse.

APPREHENSION TEST OF THE SHOULDER (CRANK TEST)[41]

The patient can be sitting, standing, or supine. The clinician places patient's shoulder in abduction and external rotation (90 degrees/90 degrees). The examiner then applies an external rotation force.

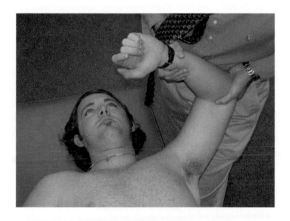

Positive sign: Patients who have experienced either dislocation or subluxation of the shoulder will become extremely apprehensive with this maneuver.

IMPINGEMENT TEST[41]

With the patient sitting, **A,** the shoulder is forcefully abducted or abducted and internally rotated, causing the greater tuberosity to press against the undersurface of the acromion. **B,** An alternative method (Hawkins-Kennedy impingement test) demonstrates the impingement sign by forcibly medially rotating the proximal humerus when the arm is forward flexed to 90 degrees.

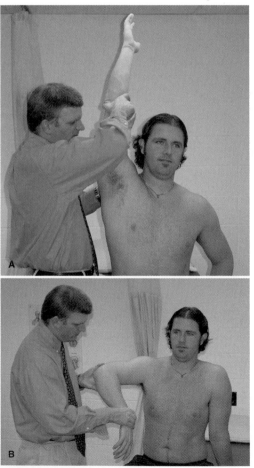

Positive sign: A positive Neer impingement sign is present if pain and its resulting facial expression are produced. A positive test indicates an impingement syndrome.

SUPRASPINATUS ISOLATION[39]

The strength of abduction of the shoulder is tested by abducting and forward flexing the arm with the forearms in internal rotation. This isolates the supraspinatus muscle, the most common area of weakness in a rotator cuff tear.

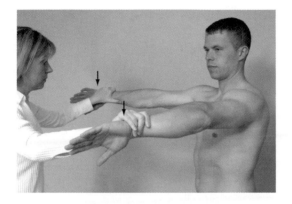

Positive sign: If weakness is demonstrated, this test is suggestive of a rotator cuff tear.

CHEST EXPANSION TEST[41]

Measured from maximal exhalation to maximal inspiration. Chest expansion is measured at **A,** the fourth lateral intercostal space, **B,** the axilla, **C,** the nipple line and **D,** the tenth rib.

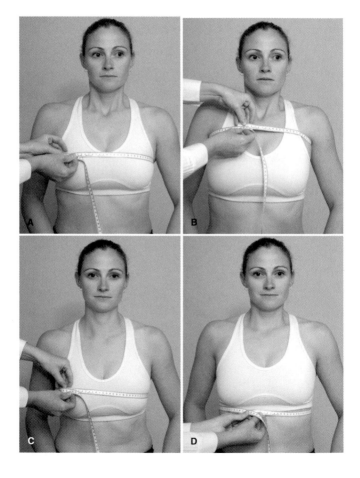

Positive sign: An expansion of less than 1 inch is indicative of forms of arthritis that can affect the spine and rib cage, most notably ankylosing spondylitis.

Knee

ANTERIOR DRAWER TEST[39,41]

The anterior drawer tests for anterior cruciate ligament deficiency.

A. In 90-degree flexion with the hip flexed 90 degrees
B. In sitting position
C. With the knee flexed approximately 90 degrees, and the proximal tibia is pulled forward
D. Flexion rotation drawer test

The therapist feels anterior shift with thumbs.

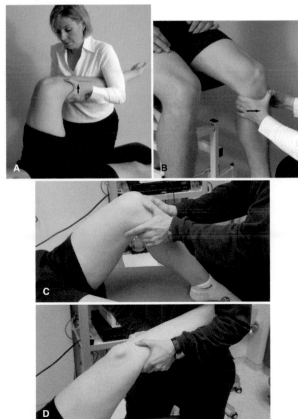

Positive sign: If excessive movement is found, the test indicates a tear of the anterior cruciate ligament.

APLEY TEST[39]

The patient is placed prone on the examining table and the knee is flexed 90 degrees. While compressing the knee, the lower leg is rotated in both directions.

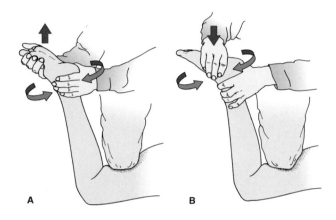

A   B

Positive sign: If this maneuver elicits pain, it is likely that a meniscal tear is present.

ELY'S TEST[39]

Ely's test tests for a tight rectus femoris. **A,** With the patient in the prone position, the examiner then flexes the leg upon the thigh. **B,** Making the heel touch the buttock.

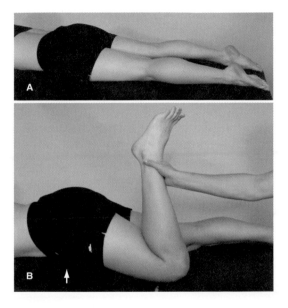

Positive sign: During flexion, the pelvis rises from the table to give a positive reaction. The reaction occurs in inflammatory or traumatic lesions.

LACHMAN'S TEST[41]

The patient lies supine on the examination table with the clinician holding the injured extremity in approximately 30 degrees of knee flexion. The clinician's outside hand holds the patient's femur firmly, while the inside hand grasps the proximal portion of the tibia The clinician slightly rotates the tibia externally while applying an anterior tibial translation force to the posterior medial portion of the tibia.

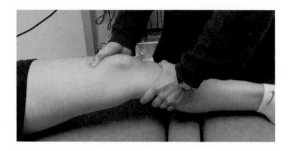

Positive sign: A positive test occurs if the translation ends in a soft end feel and the amount of laxity found is greater than that when testing the contralateral, noninjured knee. It must be noted that a false-positive result with this test can occur easily in the patient with a torn posterior cruciate ligament.

McMURRY'S TEST[41]

With the patient supine, the clinician grasps the patient's knee with the proximal hand while the distal hand grasps the foot and ankle. The clinician internally rotates the tibia on the femur using the foot as a handhold. The knee is taken into full flexion. While palpating the knee and applying a valgus stress with the proximal hand, the knee is then moved into a varus, internally rotated position while the knee is extended.

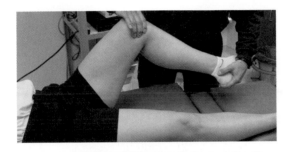

Positive sign: As the knee is flexed a second time, external tibial rotation with a valgus force can be used to implicate a tear. A click, a snap, locking, pseudolocking, or pain in either the lateral or medial joint line is indicative of a positive test for a meniscus tear.

POSTERIOR DRAWER TEST[41]

The patient is supine, and the involved hip is flexed 45 degrees and the knee flexed 80 degrees while the clinician holds the involved tibia in a neutral position. The position of 80 degrees of knee flexion is used to prevent the meniscus' ability to act as a "chock block" during this test. While using thumbs to palpate the proximal tibial plateau, the clinician gives a posteriorly-directed force onto the proximal tibia while feeling for both quantity of movement and quality of the endfeel.

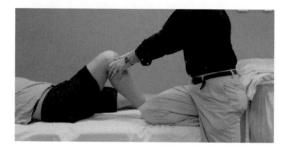

Positive sign: A positive test result would be indicated if the involved tibia moves farther posteriorly on the femur than does the uninvolved tibia. Excessive movement is indicative of a tear in the posterior cruciate ligament.

SLOCUM TEST[39]

The Slocum test assesses both anterior rotary instabilities. The patient's knee is flexed to 80 or 90 degrees, and the hip is flexed to 45 degrees. The foot is first placed in 30-degree medial rotation. The clinician sits on the patient's forefoot to hold the foot in position and draws the tibia forward.

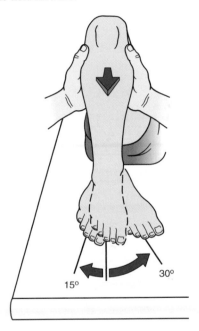

Positive sign: If the test is positive, movement occurs primarily on the lateral side of the knee. This movement is excessive relative to the unaffected side and indicates anterolateral rotary instability.

It can also indicate that other structures may have been injured to some degree, such as:

1. Anterior cruciate ligament
2. Posterolateral capsule
3. Arcuate-popliteus complex
4. Lateral collateral ligament
5. Posterior cruciate ligament
6. Iliotibial band

Hip/Pelvis

LAGUERRE'S TEST[39]

The patient is supine. To test the left sacroiliac joint, the clinician flexes, abducts, and laterally rotates the patient's left hip, applying an overpressure at the end of the ROM. The clinician must stabilize the pelvis on the opposite side by holding the opposite ASIS down. The other side is tested for comparison.

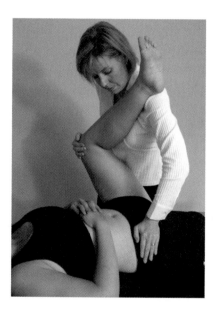

Positive sign: Pain in the sacroiliac joint constitutes a positive test. This test should be performed with caution for patients with hip pathology, because it may aggravate hip pain.

PATRICK'S TEST (FABER OR FIGURE-FOUR TEST)[53]

This tests hip or SI problems. The patient is supine with one leg extended and the test leg crossed over the extended leg just above the knee. The test leg hip is flexed, abducted, and externally rotated (FABER). Pressure is then exerted on the flexed knee.

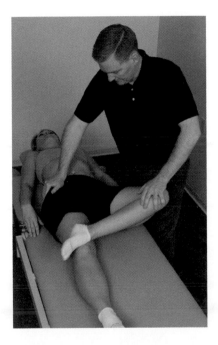

Positive sign: A positive reaction causes pain. When the test is performed in a healthy individual or in one with sciatica, pain is not produced. Discomfort is elicited in hip disorders, and in lesions of the sacroiliac ligaments at the site involved.

SLUMP TEST[53]

The patient is sitting and is asked to slump the back through the full range of thoracic and lumbar flexion and at the same time prevent the head and neck from flexing. Gentle overpressure is applied to the upper thoracic area to stretch the thoracic and lumbar spines into full flexion (**A**). As thoracic/lumbar flexion is maintained, the patient is asked to fully flex the neck, bringing the chin to the sternum. The therapist applies gentle overpressure to the fully flexed spine (**B**). As overpressure is maintained to the fully flexed spine, the patient is asked to extend one knee. The range and pain response are noted (**C**). With this position maintained, active ankle dorsiflexion is added to the knee extension and the pain response is noted (**D**). With the leg and thoracic/lumbar positions maintained with therapist overpressure, the patient is asked to move the neck into a neutral position (**E**).

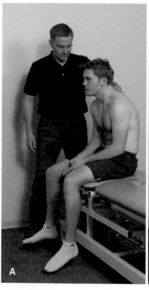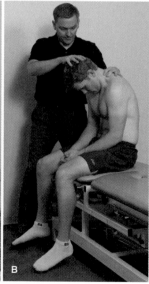

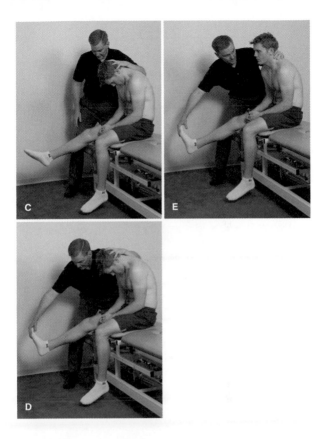

Positive sign: Positive test results are seen when lower extremity symptoms are reproduced, knee extension is limited in the slump-sit position, and when symptoms are alleviated and knee ROM is improved with a return of the neck to a neutral position.

STRAIGHT-LEG RAISING[53]

Straight-leg raising tests for the cause of leg symptoms. **A,** With the knee extended and the patient supine or seated, the hip is flexed (with the leg straight). **B,** The foot is then dorsiflexed, causing a return of symptoms; this indicates a positive test. **C,** To make the symptoms more provocative, the neck can be flexed by lifting the head at the same time as the foot is dorsiflexed.

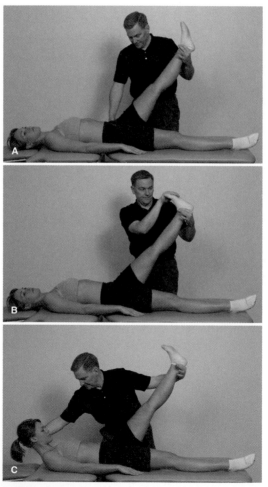

Positive sign: A positive test results in pain in the sciatic nerve distribution and suggests a disc herniation.

TRENDELENBURG TEST[39,61]

The Trendelenburg test detects weak hip abductor muscles. The patient stands and balances on one foot and then the other. Observing from behind, the therapist notes any asymmetry or change in the level of the iliac crests. **A,** Anterior view, negative test. **B,** Side view, negative test. **C,** Posterior view, positive test for a weak right gluteus medius.

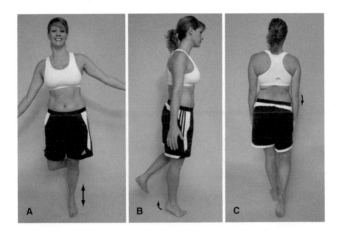

Positive sign: When the iliac crest drops on the side of the lifted leg, the hip abductor muscles on the weight-bearing side are weak. A positive test indicates gluteus medius weakness or a dislocated hip.

Spine

BACK MOVEMENTS[7,19]

Flexion: the facet joints separate or open, and in extension they compress or close.

Sidebending (lateral flexion): the facets close on the concavity of the curve and open on the convexity.

Rotation: the facets compress or close on the side toward which the rotation occurs.

Flexion from the head down: the superior vertebra rotates and translates anteriorly and the facets, lamina, or transverse processes will be felt more prominently.

Extension: the superior vertebra rotates and translates posteriorly, causing the facets, lamina, and transverse processes to be less prominent.

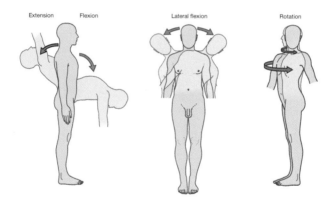

Positive sign: If a vertebra has a movement restriction, it will not move in this predicted manner. If an asymmetry in the depth of the landmarks is felt, the nature of the motion restriction from the position of the patient when the asymmetry was noted (e.g., flexion or sidebending) and the position of the landmarks can be determined.

STANDING FLEXION TEST[7]

The standing flexion test is used to determine the side of an iliosacral lesion. The patient stands with feet hip distance apart, bearing weight symmetrically. The therapist is positioned with eyes level to the posterior superior iliac spine (PSIS) and the thumbs are placed on or just under the PSIS. The patient bends forward, keeping the knees straight. The amount of cranial movement of the PSISs is observed.

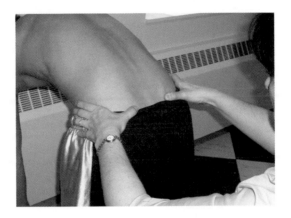

Positive sign: The test is considered positive for restricted mobility if the PSIS on one side moves more cephalad, or moves before, the one on the other side.

SACRAL FIXATION TEST (ALSO CALLED GILLET'S TEST, MARCHING TEST, OR STORK TEST)[7]

Used to determine the side of an iliosacral lesion. With the patient standing, the therapist places one thumb under the PSIS on the side being tested, with the other on the adjacent part of the sacrum. The patient is instructed to stand on one leg and flex the other hip and knee, bringing the leg towards the chest. This is repeated on each side.

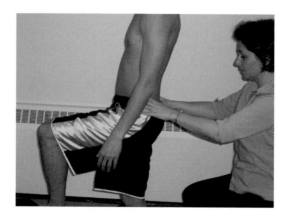

Positive sign: A test is considered positive for restricted mobility if little or no PSIS movement occurs.

LANDMARKS PALPATED FOR SYMMETRY AS PART OF THE SACROILIAC EXAMINATION[7]

During the postural and structural examination, the therapist should examine for asymmetry in the paired anatomical landmarks of the sacrum, pelvis, and lower extremity.

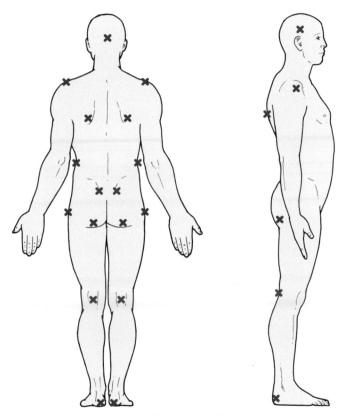

Positive sign: The absence of a leg-length discrepancy suggests the need for specific evaluation of the SI joint.

PRONE INSTABILITY TEST[7,18]

This test confirms the diagnosis of segmental spinal instability. With the patient prone on a plinth with hips at the edge and feet touching the floor, the therapist applies a posterior to anterior pressure through the lumbar spinous process to be tested (**A**). The same procedure is repeated with the patient lifting his or her feet off the floor to activate the iliocostalis and thus stabilize the segment (**B**).

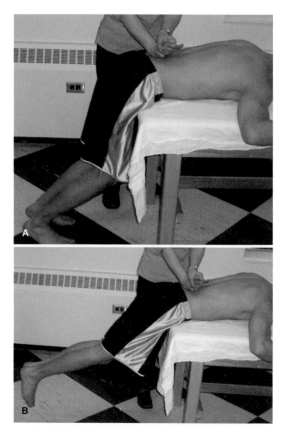

Positive sign: The test is considered positive for instability at that level if symptoms are provoked only during active muscle contraction.

Neck

POSITION TESTING OF THE CERVICAL SPINE[7]

Usually performed with the patient sitting. The patient is positioned in a neutral prone position (**A**) flexed (**B**) and an extended position, and the spinal landmarks are palpated in each position.

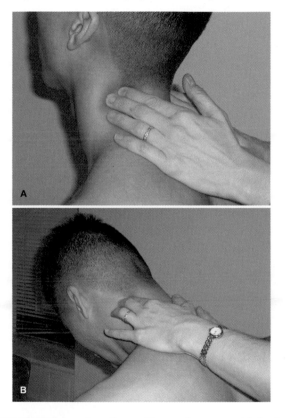

Positive sign: Determines the position and movement behavior of one vertebra relative to the vertebra directly below it.

SUPINE VERTEBRAL ARTERY TEST[7]

There are several variations of this test that determine whether extremes of movement of the cervical spine will compromise the vertebral artery and thus the cerebral circulation. All use combinations of cervical extension and rotation, with some adding traction or compression. **A,** With cervical spine rotation. **B,** With cervical spine rotation and extension. Throughout the procedure the therapist carefully watches and questions the patient for any occurrence of symptoms.

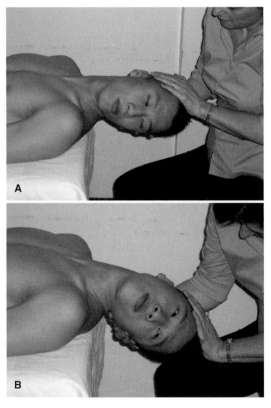

Positive sign: If any symptoms occur, the test is positive and high-velocity or maintained end-range techniques of the cervical spine are contraindicated.

SPURLING'S TEST[7]

Spurling's test involves cervical sidebending and extension together with axial compression or overpressure.

With the patient sitting, the therapist rotates the head to one side, side bends to the same side, and extends. Gentle overpressure is applied by the therapist's hand on the patient's temple.

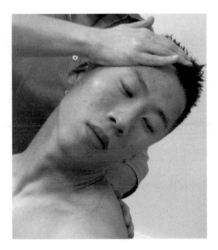

Positive sign: Reproduction of symptoms in the neck or arm corresponding to the side of bending constitutes a positive test. When symptoms occur with sidebending away from the side of pain, an intervertebral disc dysfunction is implicated. If pain is reproduced with lateral flexion toward the side of pain, foraminal encroachment is thought to be the cause.

Hand/Wrist/Thumb

FINKELSTEIN'S TEST TO DETECT TENOSYNOVITIS OF THE THUMB OR DE QUERVAIN'S SYNDROME[15]

The patient makes a fist with the thumb inside the palm. The therapist holds the forearm steady and deviates the wrist ulnarly.

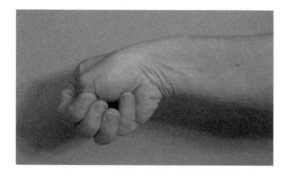

Positive sign: Pain indicates De Quervain's tendonitis of the wrist.

PHALEN'S TEST[39]

Clinical examination for carpal tunnel syndrome includes Phalen's test.

The patient holds the backs of the hands together by flexing the wrists at 90 degrees and holds for 60 seconds.

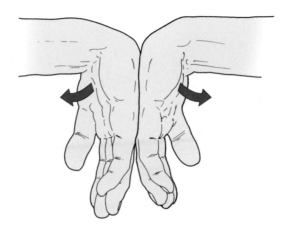

Positive sign: A positive test is indicated by tingling in the thumb, index finger, and middle and lateral half of the ring finger and is indicative of carpal tunnel syndrome caused by pressure on the median nerve.

Nerves

TINEL'S TEST AND SIGN[3,7,39]

Tinel's test is used to detect Tinel's sign, which is a hyperirritability or response to mechanical inputs such as tapping, and is thought to be indicative of nerve injury. Examples: **A,** Anterior tibial branch of deep peroneal nerve. **B,** Posterior tibial nerve. **C,** Detecting carpel tunnel.

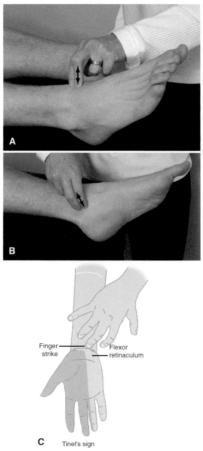

Positive sign: A tingling sensation in the distal end of a limb when percussion is made over the site of a divided nerve can indicate a partial lesion or the beginning of regeneration of the nerve.

PLANTAR OR BABINSKI'S REFLEX[37]

The therapist strokes from the heel to the ball of the foot along the lateral sole, then across the ball of the foot. Also called Babinski's sign. **A,** Normal. This action will cause the toes to flex. **B,** Developmental or pathologic issues. Babinski's sign in response to the same stimulus.

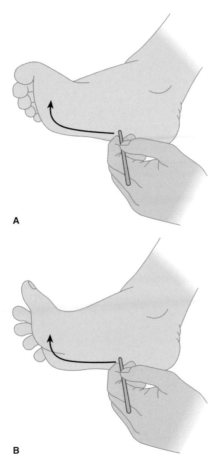

A

B

Positive sign: In people with corticospinal tract lesions or in infants less than 7 months old, the great toe extends. Although the other toes may fan out, as shown, movement of the toes other than the great toe is not required for Babinski's sign.

Special Neurological Tests[57]

Test	Description	Response	Clinical Importance
Babinski's sign (extensor plantar)	Plantar surface of foot is stroked with key or fingernail in a sweeping motion from posterior and lateral border toward ball of foot	Extension of great toe, with or without fanning of other toes	Indicates upper motor neuron lesion
Oppenheim reflex	Anterior border of tibia is stroked	Presence of Babinski's sign	If Babinski's sign present, indicates upper motor neuron lesion
Hoffmann's sign	Distal phalanx of index, middle, or ring finger is subjected to rapid, gentle stroking	Reflexive flexion of thumb distal interphalangeal joint or distal interphalangeal joint of any other finger not struck	If present, indicates upper motor neuron lesion
Abdominal reflex	Upper or lower abdominal musculature is gently stroked	Motion of umbilicus toward stroking	Reduction or absence indicates upper motor neuron damage or involvement of pertinent spinal level reflexes (T7–9, upper abdominal region; T11–12, lower abdominal region)
Romberg's sign	Subject stands with feet close together and then closes eyes	Subject increases sway or falls with eyes closed	Indicates dorsal (sensory) column disease or pathology
Rapidly alternating movements	Subject performs rapid forearm pronation and supination or ankle plantar flexion and dorsiflexion	Inability to perform movement (dysdiadochokinesia)	Indicates ipsilateral cerebellar dysfunction, especially lateral hemispheres
Finger to nose	Subject extends finger away from face and then toward nose, and repeats this movement	Subject able to perform movement smoothly, correctly estimating distances and location	If movement is not smooth or there is overshooting or undershooting of movement, then may indicate cerebellar dysfunction (asynergy)

Common Imaging Techniques[16]

Test	Description	Type of Tissue
Magnetic resonance imaging (MRI)	Uses radiofrequency to view structures; considered superior to CT for central nervous system (CNS) tissues	CNS, organs, soft tissue, cartilage
Computed tomography (CT)	Provides cross sections of tissues 100× more sensitive than radiographs	Soft tissues, stress fractures, tumors, bleeding
Myelogram	Radiograph taken of a given area following a radiopaque injection that allows for illumination of specific structures	Spinal cord, meninges, specific cells in bone marrow
Radiograph	Picture using high-speed electrons that can penetrate most objects	Bony structure integrity, certain masses and tumors
Electrocardiogram (ECG)	A record of the heart's electrical activity	Heart
Bone scan	CT performed of a given area following a radiopaque injection that allows for illumination of specific structures	Stress fractures, osteoarthritis, bone activity levels
Mammogram	A radiograph of the soft tissues of the breast	Breast tissue, certain masses
Colonoscopy	Visualization into the colon	Colon
Endoscopy	Visualization into a specific body cavity	Bronchoscope (upper respiratory)
		Laparoscope (abdomen)
		Gastroscope (upper gastrointestinal)
Venogram, phlebogram	A radiograph of a vein is taken following injection of a radiopaque injection into the vein	Veins

Guidelines For Referral[24,39]

Immediate medical attention	Patient with anginal pain not relieved in 20 min
	Patient with angina who has nausea, vomiting, profuse sweating
	Diabetic patient demonstrating signs of confusion, lethargy, or changes in mental alertness and function
	Patient with bowel or bladder incontinence and/or saddle anesthesia secondary to cauda equina lesion
	Patient in anaphylactic shock
Medical attention necessary	
General systemic	Unknown cause
	Lack of significant objective neuromusculoskeletal signs and symptoms
	Lack of expected progress with physical therapy treatment
	Development of constitutional symptoms or associated signs and symptoms over the course of treatment
	Discovery of significant past medical history (PMH) unknown to physician
	Changes in health status that persist 7–10 days beyond expected time period
	Patient who is jaundiced and has not been diagnosed or treated
	Changes in size, shape, tenderness, and consistency of lymph nodes in more than one area, which persist more than 4 wk; painless, enlarged lymph nodes
For women	Low back, hip, pelvic, groin, or sacroiliac symptoms without known etiology and in the presence of constitutional symptoms
	Symptoms correlated with menses
	Any spontaneous uterine bleeding after menopause
	For pregnant women: vaginal bleeding, elevated blood pressure, increased Braxton Hicks contractions during exercise
Vital signs (report these findings)	Persistent rise or fall of blood pressure
	Blood pressure evaluation in any woman taking birth control pills (should be closely monitored by her physician)
	Pulse amplitude that fades with inspiration and strengthens with expiration
	Pulse increase more than 20 beats/min lasting more than 3 min after rest or changing position
	Difference between systolic and diastolic measurements of more than 40 mm Hg in pulse pressure
	Persistent low-grade (or higher) fever, especially associated with constitutional symptoms, most commonly sweats
Cardiac	Angina at rest
	Anginal pain not relieved in 20 min
	More than three sublingual nitroglycerin tablets required to gain relief
	Nitroglycerin does not relieve anginal pain
	Rest does not relieve angina
	Angina continues to increase in intensity after stimulus (e.g., cold, stress, exertion) has been eliminated
	Changes in pattern of angina
	Abnormally severe chest pain
	Patient has nausea, vomiting
	Anginal pain radiates to jaw or left arm
	Upper back feels abnormally cool, sweaty, or moist to touch
	Patient has any doubts about his or her condition

Cancer	Early warning sign or signs of cancer: seven early warning signs plus two additional signs pertinent to the physical therapy examination; proximal muscle weakness and change in deep tendon reflexes
	All soft-tissue lumps that persist or grow, whether painful or painless
	Any women presenting with chest, breast, axillary, or shoulder pain of unknown etiology, especially in the presence of a positive medical history (self or family) of cancer
	Bone pain, especially on weight bearing, that persists more than 1 wk and is worse at night
Pulmonary	Shoulder pain that is aggravated by supine positioning
	Shoulder, chest (thorax) pain that subsides with autosplinting (lying on the painful side)
	For the patient with asthma: signs of asthma or bronchial activity during exercise
Genitourinary	Abnormal urinary constituents, e.g., change in color, odor, amount, flow of urine
	Any amount of blood in urine
Musculoskeletal	Symptoms that seem out of proportion to the injury, or symptoms persisting beyond the expected time for the nature of the injury
	Severe or chronic back pain accompanied by constitutional symptoms, especially fever
Precautions/ contraindications to therapy	Uncontrolled chronic heart failure or pulmonary edema
	Active myocarditis
	Resting heart rate > 120 or 130 beats/min
	Resting systolic rate > 180–200 beats/min
	Resting diastolic rate > 105–110 beats/min
	Moderate dizziness, near-syncope
	Marked dyspnea
	Unusual fatigue
	Unsteadiness
	Loss of palpable pulse
	Postoperative posterior calf pain
	(For the patient with diabetes): chronically unstable blood sugar levels must be stabilized (normal: 80–120 mg/dL; "safe": 100–250 mg/dl)

Evaluation, Diagnosis, and Prognosis

Evaluating Cranial Nerves[4,37]

#	Name	Function	Tests	Significant Findings
I	Olfactory	Smell	Odor recognition (unilateral)	Lack of odor perception on one or both sides
II	Optic	Vision	Visual acuity; peripheral vision; papillary light reflex	Reduced vision
III	Oculomotor	Moves eyes up, down, medially; raises upper eyelid; constricts pupil	Extraocular eye movements; papillary light reflex	Impairment of one or more eye movements or disconjugate gaze; papillary dilation; ptosis
IV	Trochlear	Moves eye medially and down	Extraocular eye movements	Impairment of one or more eye movements or disconjugate gaze
V	Trigeminal	Facial sensation, chewing, sensation from temporomandibular joint	Sensation above eye, between eye and mouth, below mouth to angle of jaw; palpation of contraction of masseter and temporalis muscles	Reduced sensation in one or more divisions of the fifth nerve; impaired jaw reflex; reduced strength in masseter and temporalis muscles
VI	Abducens	Abducts eye	Extraocular eye movements	Reduced eye abduction
VII	Facial	Facial expression, closes eyes, tears, salivation, and taste	Facial expression; taste of anterior two thirds of tongue	Weakness of upper or lower face or eye closure; reduced taste perception (salty, sweet, bitter, sour)
VIII	Acoustic	Sensation of head position relative to gravity and head movement; hearing	Auditory and vestibular	Reduced hearing; impaired balance
IX	Glossopharyngeal	Swallowing, salivation, and taste	Gag reflex; speech (phonation); swallowing	Impaired reflex; dysarthria; dysphagia
X	Vagus	Regulates viscera, swallowing, speech, and taste	Phonation; coughing; gag reflex	Hoarseness; weak cough; impaired reflex
XI	Accessory	Elevates shoulders, turns head	Resisted head; shoulder shrug	Weakness of trapezius and sternocleidomastoid
XII	Hypoglossal	Moves tongue	Tongue protrusion	Deviation, atrophy, or fasciculations of tongue

Spinal Disorder Diagnoses[7]

Derangement syndrome   One of the major categories of the McKenzie classification system, characterized by anatomical disruption of the structures of the intervertebral joints.

Dysfunction syndrome   One of the major categories of the McKenzie classification system, characterized by pain that results from mechanical deformation of structurally impaired soft tissue after degeneration, trauma, or inflammation.

Limb-length inequality (LLI)   A difference in length between the two lower extremities. In anatomical LLI, one of the bones of the lower extremity is shortened. In functional LLI, shortening of one of the lower extremities occurs without shortening of the bones.

Neurogenic claudication   A condition characterized by aggravation of neurological signs and symptoms, such as pain, paresthesia, and lower extremity cramping with ambulation, or by increasing lumbar lordosis of the spine. Symptoms improve with a change in posture.

Postural syndrome   One of the major categories of the McKenzie classification system, characterized by pain that results from maintenance of poor posture.

Radiculopathy   Irritation of a nerve root at any level of the spine.

Spinal stenosis   Narrowing of the spinal canal or intervertebral foramina because of bony or soft tissue encroachment. Where the space between the spinal cord or nerve roots and the vertebral elements is compromised.

Spondylolisthesis   Translation of vertebra forward in the sagittal plane with respect to an adjacent vertebra.

Spondylosis   A bilateral defect in the pars interarticularis of a vertebra that decreases the ability of the posterior elements to stabilize the motion segment.

Whiplash-associated disorders (WAD)   Bony or soft-tissue injuries of the neck and related areas that occur after a rear or side motor vehicle collision, in which the neck is subjected to acceleration-deceleration energy transfer.

Connective Tissue Dysfunction Diagnoses[7]

Ankylosing spondylitis (AS)   A form of inflammatory arthritis that has a predilection for the sacroiliac joints, axial spine, and ligamentous/tendinous insertions.

Arteritis   Inflammation of the arteries.

Arthralgia   Joint pain.

Arthritis   Encompasses over 100 types of rheumatic diseases, but the literal translation means inflammation of the joint.

Avascular necrosis   Necrosis of bone caused by ischemia.

Baker's cyst   A cystic swelling within the popliteal space posterior to the knee as a result of mechanical irritation or synovial inflammation.

Boutonnière deformity   A finger deformity with flexion at the proximal interphalangeal (PIP) joint and hyperextension at the distal interphalangeal (DIP) joint.

Bursitis   Inflammation at the bursa, which may be due to trauma, frictional forces, or rheumatic disease.

Dactylitis   Inflammation of a finger or toe.

Dermatomyositis (DM)   Diffuse inflammatory disease of striated muscle that leads to symmetric proximal muscle weakness with a dermatological component.

Discoid lupus   A form of lupus that involves skin disease with distinctive erythematous scaly plaques.

Effusion   Excess fluid in the joint resulting from joint irritation or inflammation of the synovium.

Enthesitis   Inflammation where ligaments and tendons attach to bone.

Gout   A disease characterized by an acute episode of arthritis resulting from the deposition of uric acid crystals at the joint or in surrounding tissues.

Hyperuricemia   Abnormal amount of uric acid in the blood.

Inflammatory arthritis   Systemic arthritis that involves inflammation of the synovium of the joint.

Leukopenia   Abnormal decrease in white blood cells (WBCs).

Livedo reticularis   A semipermanent bluish mottling of the skin of the legs and hands.

Lupus   A chronic inflammatory autoimmune disease that may affect the skin, joints, and internal organs.

Myositis   Inflammatory disease of striated muscle.

Nephritis   Inflammation of the kidney.

Pannus   Excessive proliferation of synovial and granulation tissue that invades joint surfaces.

Panniculitis   Inflamed condition of a layer of fatty connective tissue in the anterior wall of the abdomen.

Pauciarticular   Involvement of few joints.

Pericarditis   Inflammation of the pericardium.

Pleurisy   Inflammation of the pleura.

Polymyalgia rheumatica (PMR)   Condition characterized by stiffness and pain at the shoulder girdle without weakness; usually seen in women over 50 years of age in conjunction with an elevated erythrocyte sedimentation rate (ESR).

Polymyositis (PM)   Diffuse inflammatory disease of striated muscle that leads to symmetric proximal muscle weakness.

Pseudogout   Synovitis caused by the deposition of calcium pyrophosphate dehydrate crystals resulting in arthritis; articular chondrocalcinosis.

Psoriatic arthritis (PA)   A spondyloarthropathy with concomitant psoriasis.

Purpura   Condition characterized by hemorrhage into the skin.

Raynaud's phenomenon   An intermittent vasoconstriction of the distal small arteries, arterioles, and capillaries that results in blanching, erythema, and cyanosis of the hands.

Reactive arthritis   Spondyloarthropathy with enteric or venereal infectious trigger.

Reiter's syndrome (RS)   Triad of arthritis, conjunctivitis, and urethritis.

Rheumatoid arthritis (RA)   Systemic disease characterized by inflammation of the joint synovium.

Sclerodactyly   Sclerosis and tapering of the fingers in progressive systemic sclerosis.

Scleroderma (Sc)   A chronic disease of unknown etiology that causes sclerosis of the skin and organs (gastrointestinal tract, heart, lungs, and kidneys) and arthritis.

Sjögren's syndrome (SS)   Disease of the lacrimal and parotid glands resulting in dry eyes and mouth; frequently occurs with RA, systemic lupus erythematosus (SLE), and SS.

Spondyloarthropathy   Inflammation of the spine and sacroiliac joints. Describes a category of diseases including ankylosing spondylitis, reactive arthritis/Reiter's syndrome, and psoriatic arthritis, and all may include inflammatory bowel disease as well.

Synovitis   Inflammation of the synovium.

Systemic lupus erythematosus (SLE)   Systemic inflammatory disease characterized by small vessel vasculitis and a diverse clinical presentation.

Systemic sclerosis (SSc)   A class of scleroderma, which is a chronic disease of unknown etiology that causes sclerosis of the skin and organs (GI tract, heart, lungs, and kidneys) and arthritis.

Tenosynovitis   Inflammation of the synovial lining of the tendon sheaths.

Uveitis   Inflammation of the iris, ciliary body, and choroids, or the entire uvea.

Vasculitis   Inflammation of the blood or lymph vessels.

Xerostomia   Dry mouth.

Xerophthalmia   Dry eyes.

Examples of Fractures[7]

Fractures	Definition	Examples
Avulsion fractures		
	Fractures caused by a tendon or ligament pulling off a small piece of bone to which it is attached.	
Boxer's fracture		
	A fracture of fourth and/or fifth metacarpal often seen after the patient strikes an object or person.	
Closed fracture[33]		
	A fracture without a break in the overlying skin.	

Closed, nondisplaced

Continued

Fractures	Definition	Examples

Colles' fracture[8]

A metaphyseal fracture of the distal radius that is dorsally angulated.

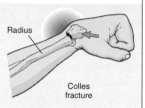

Radius

Colles fracture

Comminuted fracture[33]

A fracture that forms more than two pieces of bone.

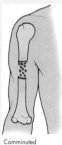

Comminuted (fragmented)

Compression fracture[8]

A fracture in which cancellous bone collapses and compresses on itself. Typically this occurs in the vertebral bodies.

Compression fracture

Delayed union

Progression of healing of a fracture that is slower than average.

Fracture

A break in a bone.

Fractures	Definition	Examples

Greenstick fracture[33]

A fracture through only one side of a bone. These fractures are common in children.

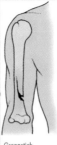

Greenstick

Impaction fracture[33]

A fracture in which a bony fragment, generally cortical, is forced or impacted into cancellous bone. Typically this occurs at the ends of long bones.

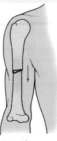

Impacted

Irregularly shaped bones

Bones such as those in the jaw or the spinal column that are of various shapes, examples of which are the mandible and the vertebrae.

Linear fracture

A fracture that runs parallel to the long axis of a bone.

Malunions

Fractures that have united with angulation or rotation to a degree that gives a displeasing appearance or adversely affects function.

Continued

Fractures	Definition	Examples
Oblique fracture[33]	A fracture at approximately 30 degrees to the long axis of the bone.	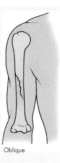 Oblique
Open fracture[33]	A fracture in which the skin is broken, exposing the fracture site to the external environment.	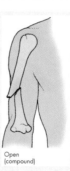 Open (compound)
Osteomyelitis	Inflammation of the bone caused by a pathological organism.	
Pseudoarthrosis	A false joint that develops at the site of a fracture	
Stress fracture	A fracture caused by repeated, prolonged, or abnormal stress.	
Torus fracture	A fracture that warps but does not completely break one side of the cortex of the bone, also known as a buckle fracture. This fracture is most commonly seen in children.	
Transverse fracture	A fracture perpendicular to the long axis of the bone.	

Polyneuropathies[7]

Acute inflammatory demyelinating polyneuropathy (AIDP) Most common variant of Guillain-Barré syndrome (GBS). An autoimmune disease directed against myelin.

Acute motor axonal neuropathy (AMAN) A variant of GBS that primarily affects the motor nerve axons.

Acute motor sensory axonal neuropathy (AMSAN) A variant of GBS that primarily affects the motor and sensory nerve axons.

Alcoholic neuropathy Decreased nerve functioning caused by damage from excessive drinking of alcohol.

Allodynia The sensation of pain in response to sensory stimulation that is usually not painful.

Autonomic neuropathy Damage to nerves that regulate autonomic functions, including blood pressure, heart rate, bowel and bladder emptying, and digestion.

Charcot-Marie-Tooth (CMT) disease A group of inherited, slowly progressive disorders that result from progressive damage to nerves. Symptoms include numbness and muscle atrophy that first occur in the feet and legs and then in the hands and arms.

Chronic inflammatory demyelinating polyradiculoneuropathy (CIDP) An autoimmune disease directed against myelin or Schwann cell antigens that causes slowly progressive or relapsing motor and/or sensory symptoms in more than one limb, developing over at least 8 weeks.

Diabetic neuropathy A common complication of diabetes mellitus in which nerves are damaged as a result of hyperglycemia (high blood sugar levels).

Guillain-Barré syndrome (GBS) An autoimmune disease directed against myelin that causes progressive muscle weakness or paralysis over a few days, which often starts a few days after resolution of an infectious illness.

Mononeuropathy Dysfunction of a single nerve or nerve group.

Peripheral neuropathy Dysfunction of the peripheral nerves.

Polyneuropathy Generally a bilateral, symmetrical disturbance of peripheral nerve function.

Lymphatic System Disorders Diagnoses[7]

Cellulitis   Diffuse acute inflammation of the skin and subcutaneous tissue.

Filariasis   Disease caused by the presence of parasitic worms that occlude the lymphatic channels.

Hyperkeratosis   A condition marked by thickening of the outer layer of the skin that can result from normal use, chronic inflammation, or genetic disorders.

Lymphangitis   Inflammation of one or more lymphatic vessels.

Lymphedema   A disorder characterized by swelling caused by accumulation of lymph in soft tissues.

Subcutaneous fibrosclerosis   Hardening below the skin caused by abnormal formation of fibrous tissue.

Spinal Cord Injuries

EXAMPLES OF NONPROGRESSIVE SPINAL DISORDERS[7]

Anterior cord syndrome   Destruction of the anterior portion of the spinal cord that results in a pattern of impairments characterized by complete loss of motor function and some loss of light touch and temperature sensation, with sparing of proprioception and discriminative touch.

Autonomic dysreflexia (AD)   A serious, life-threatening emergency condition that is the result of an uncontrolled autonomic response to a noxious stimulus from either an external or an internal (visceral) source.

Brown-Séquard syndrome   Damage to one half of the spinal cord, resulting in a pattern of impairments characterized by ipsilateral proprioceptive and motor loss and contralateral loss of pain and temperature sensation.

Cauda equina syndrome   Damage to the lumbar or sacral nerve roots, resulting in sensory loss and flaccid paralysis below the injury level.

Central cord syndrome   Injury to the central portion of the spinal cord, resulting in a pattern of impairments characterized by weakness more severe in upper extremities (UEs) than in lower extremities (LEs), with sparing of sacral sensation.

Central pattern generators   Neural circuits within the spinal cord that are able to produce.

Paraplegia Loss of function in the thoracic, lumbar, or sacral segments of the spinal cord, resulting in sparing of UE function but possible impairments in the trunk, pelvis, and LEs, depending on the segment of the lesion.

Pressure ulcer A common complication of spinal cord injury (SCI) characterized by ischemic ulceration of soft tissue as a result of unrelieved pressure and shearing forces.

Quadriplegia SCI affecting all four extremities; synonym for tetraplegia.

Spasticity A disorder that can occur below the level of SCI characterized by velocity-dependent hypertonia, resulting from a combination of multiple changes in neural control and muscle properties.

Spinal cord injury (SCI) Damage to the neurological components of the spinal cord as the result of primary or secondary effects of disease or trauma.

Tetraplegia Loss of function because of damage of the neural elements in the cervical segments of the spinal cord, resulting in impairment or loss of motor and/or sensory function involving the upper extremities, as well as more caudal functions.

KEY TERMS IMPORTANT TO THE ASSESSMENT OF SPINAL CORD INJURY[62]

Complete injury The absence of sensory and motor function in the lowest sacral segments.

Incomplete injury Preservation of motor or sensory function below the neurological level of injury that includes the lowest sacral segments.

Motor index score Calculated by adding the muscle scores of each key muscle group; a total score of 100 is possible.

Motor level The most caudal key muscle group that is graded 3/5 or greater with the segments cephalad graded normal (5/5) strength.

Neurological level of injury The most caudal level at which both motor and sensory modalities are intact.

Sacral sparing Presence of motor function (voluntary external anal sphincter contraction) or sensory function (light touch, pinprick at S4/5 dermatome, or anal sensation on rectal examination) in the lowest sacral segments.

Sensory index score Calculated by adding the scores for each dermatome; a total score of 112 is possible for each pinprick and light touch.

Sensory level The most caudal dermatome to have normal sensation for both pinprick and light touch on both sides.

Zone of partial preservation All segments below the neurological level of injury, with preservation of motor or sensory findings; used only in complete SCI.

(Sisto, SA: *Spinal cord injuries: management and rehabilitation*, St. Louis, 2009, Mosby).

ASIA Impairment Scale

Grade	Impairment
A = Complete	No motor or sensory function is preserved in the sacral segments S4 and S5.
B = Incomplete	Sensory but not motor function is preserved below the neurologic level and includes the sacral segments S4 and S5.
C = Incomplete	Motor function is preserved below the neurologic level, and more than half of key muscles below the neurologic level have a muscle grade less than 3.
D = Incomplete	Motor function is preserved below the neurologic level, and at least half of key muscles below the neurologic level have a muscle grade of 3 or more.
E = Normal	Motor and sensory functions are normal.

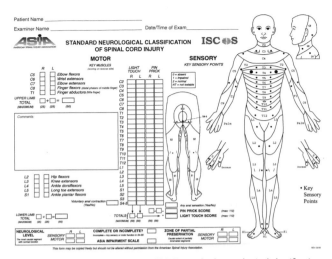

American Spinal Injury Association (ASIA) standard neurological classification of spinal cord injury (Courtesy American Spinal Injury Association, Atlanta, GA, 2006) (www.asia-spinalinjury.org)

Indications for Joint Mobilization[7]

Symptom Characteristics	Examination Findings
Mechanical origin	Symptoms are aggravated by certain movements or postures and are relieved by rest or other positions
Diminished ROM	Loss of active or passive osteokinematic movement found on examination of ROM, PPIVM, and position testing
Joint hypomobility	Diminished arthrokinematic movement determined by diminished passive mobility (PA) and position testing
Joint asymmetry	Asymmetrical movement at individual joints as determined by PPIVM and position testing
Tissue texture abnormality	Abnormal resistances to movement as a result of pain, spasm, trigger points, or thickened and stiff soft tissues overlying the joint
Pain	Neuromusculoskeletal pain on movement, palpation, and elicited by provocation tests

ROM, Range of motion; *PPIVM*, passive physiological intervertebral mobility; *PA*, posterior to anterior.

The ABCDs of Skin Cancer[16]

	Descriptor	Parameters
A	Asymmetry	A melanoma lesion cannot be "folded in half"; in other words, the lesion does not have equal right and left sections or top and bottom sections.
B	Border	Benign lesions have a sharp, distinct border that can be traced easily, whereas malignant lesions may have borders that can fade off and be difficult to trace.
C	Color	Benign lesions have a uniform tan, brown, or black color, whereas malignant lesions may have variegated or multiple (i.e., red, white, and blue) color patterns. In addition, a sudden darkening in color or spreading into normal skin suggests a malignant lesion.
D	Diameter	Benign lesions usually have a diameter of less than 6 mm, whereas malignant lesions usually have a diameter greater than 6 mm.

Skin, Hand, and Nail Infections[24,25]

Type of Infection	Example	Method of Transmission
Bacterial		
Impetigo contagiosa[58]		Contagious
Pyoderma[63]		Contagious

Type of Infection	Example	Method of Transmission
Folliculitis (pimple, boil)[33]	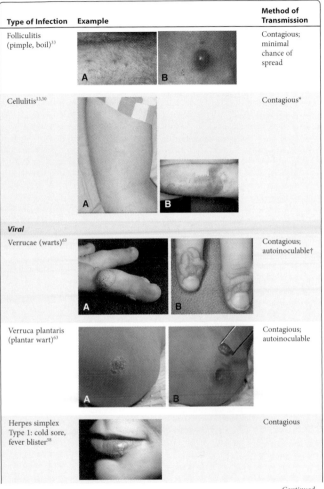	Contagious; minimal chance of spread
Cellulitis[13,50]		Contagious*
Viral		
Verrucae (warts)[63]		Contagious; autoinoculable†
Verruca plantaris (plantar wart)[63]		Contagious; autoinoculable
Herpes simplex Type 1: cold sore, fever blister[58]		Contagious

Continued

Type of Infection	Example	Method of Transmission
Varicella zoster virus (herpes zoster; shingles)[5,43]		Contagious; chickenpox can occur in anyone not previously exposed
Fungal		
Tinea corporis (ringworm)[68,27]		Person-to-person Animal-to-person Inanimate object-to-person
Tinea capitis (affects scalp)[13,27]	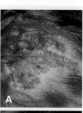	Person-to-person Animal-to-person
Tinea cruris (jock itch)		Person-to-person
Tinea pedis (athlete's foot)[35]		Transmission to other people rare despite general opinion to the contrary

Type of Infection	Example	Method of Transmission
Other		
Scabies[58]		Person-to-person; sexually transmitted during birth from colonized vaginal to neonatal oropharynx Inanimate object-to-person
Lice[43,13]		Same as scabies

*Technically, cellulitis is contagious, but from a practical point of view the chances of this spreading are very low and would require a susceptible host, e.g., an open cut on the therapist's hand coming in contact with blood or pus from the client's open wound.

†Capable of spreading infection from one's own body by scratching.

Common Causes of Skin and Nail Bed Changes[24]

Skin/Nail Bed Changes	Possible Causes
SKIN CHANGES	
Dermatitis	Pulmonary malignancy, allergic reaction
Loss of turgor or elasticity	Dehydration
Rash	Viruses (chickenpox, measles, fifth disease)
	Systemic conditions (meningitis, lupus, hives, rosacea)
	Sexually transmitted diseases
	Lyme disease
	Parasites (e.g., lice, scabies)
	Reaction to chemicals, medications, food
	Malignancy, neoplastic syndromes
Hemorrhage (petechiae, ecchymosis, NSAIDs purpura)	Anticoagulants (heparin, coumadin/warfarin, aspirin)
	Hemophilia
	Thrombocytopenia (low platelet level) and anything that can cause thrombocytopenia
	Neoplasm; paraneoplastic syndrome
	Domestic violence
	Aging

Continued

Skin/Nail Bed Changes	Possible Causes
Skin color	Jaundice (yellow, green, orange): hepatitis, chronic renal failure (yellow-brown) Cyanosis (pale, blue): anxiety, hypothermia, lung disease, congestive heart disease, venous obstruction Rubor (dusky red): arterial insufficiency Sunburn (red): radiation recall or radiation dermatitis Tan, black, blue: skin cancer
Hyperpigmentation	Addison's disease, ACTH-producing tumors Sarcoidosis Pregnancy Leukemia Hemochromatosis Celiac sprue (malabsorption) Scleroderma Chronic renal failure Hereditary (nonpathognomic) Low-dose radiation
Café-au-lait (hyperpigmentation)	Neurofibromatosis (more than five lesions) Albright's syndrome Urticaria pigmentosa (less than five lesions)
Hypopigmentation (vitiligo)	Albinism Sun exposure Steroid injections Hyperthyroidism Stomach cancer Pernicious anemia Diabetes mellitus Autoimmune diseases High-dose radiation
Xanthomas	Disorders of lipid metabolism Primary biliary cirrhosis Diabetes mellitus (uncontrolled)
Mongolian spots	Blue-black discoloration: normal in certain groups of people
NAIL BED CHANGES	
Onycholysis	Graves' disease, psoriasis, reactive arthritis, nail picking
Beau's lines	Acute systemic illness Chemotherapy Peripheral vascular disease (PVD) Eating disorders Cirrhosis (chronic alcohol use) Recent heart attack Local trauma
Koilonychia	Congenital or hereditary Hypochromic anemia Iron deficiency Diabetes mellitus (chronic, uncontrolled) Psoriasis Syphilis Rheumatic fever Thyroid dysfunction
Splinter hemorrhages	Heart attack Bacterial endocarditis Vasculitis Renal failure Any systemic insult

Skin/Nail Bed Changes	Possible Causes
Leukonychia	Acquired or congenital Acquired: hypocalcemia, hypochromic anemia, Hodgkin's disease, renal failure, malnutrition, heart attack, hepatic cirrhosis, arsenic poisoning
Paronychia	Fungal infection Bacterial infection
Digital clubbing	Acute: pulmonary abscess, malignancy, polycythemia, paraneoplastic syndrome Chronic: COPD, cystic fibrosis, congenital heart defects, cor pulmonale
Absent or underdeveloped nail bed(s)	Nail-patella-syndrome (NPS) Congenital
Pitting	Psoriasis

ACTH, Adrenocorticotropic hormone; *NSAIDS,* nonsteroidal antiinflammatory drugs.

Hand and Nail Bed Assessment[24]

Observe the Hands for:	Example
Palmar erythema[23]	
Tremor (e.g., liver flap or asterixis)[24]	 Arm extended Wrist dorsiflexed Hand "flap"
Pallor of palmar creases (anemia, GI malabsorption)[20]	
Palmar xanthomas (lipid deposits on palms of hands; hyperlipidemia, diabetes)[36]	

Observe the Hands for:	Example
Turgor (lift skin on back of hands; suggests hydration status)[10]	
Edema[32]	

Observe the Fingers and Toenails for:	
Color (capillary refill time, Terry's nails)[27]	
With Terry's nails, the nail bed is white with only a narrow zone of pink at the distal end.	
Shape and curvature	
Clubbing[20]	

Crohn's disease or cardiac/cyanosis

Lung (cancer, hypoxia, cystic fibrosis)

Ulcerative colitis

Biliary cirrhosis

Present at birth (harmless)

Neoplasm

GI involvement

- Nicotine stains
- Splinter hemorrhages
- Leukonychia (whitening of nail plate with bands, lines, or white spots; inherited or acquired from malnutrition from eating disorders, alcoholism, or cancer treatment; myocardial infarction, renal failure, poison, anxiety)
- Koilonychia ("spoon nails"; congenital or hereditary, iron deficiency anemia, thyroid problem, syphilis, rheumatic fever)

Observe the Hands for:	Example
• Beau's lines; decreased production of the nail by the matrix caused by acute illness or systemic insult such as chemotherapy for cancer; recent myocardial infarction, chronic alcohol abuse, or eating disorders; this can also occur in isolated nail beds from local trauma	
• Adhesion to the nail bed; look for onycholysis (loosening of nail plate from distal edge inward; Graves' disease, psoriasis, reactive arthritis, obsessive compulsive behavior: "nail pickers")	
• Pitting (psoriasis, eczema, alopecia areata)	
• Thinning/thickening	

Common Variations in Nail Shape[33]

Nail Shape	Clinical Findings		Significance
Normal	Angle of 160° between the nail plate and the proximal nail fold Nail surface slightly convex Nail base firm when palpated		Normal finding
Clubbing			
Early clubbing	Straightening of angle between the nail plate and the proximal nail fold to 180° Nail base spongy when palpated		Hypoxia Lung cancer
Late clubbing	Angle between the nail plate and the proximal nail fold exceeds 180° Nail base visibly edematous and spongy when palpated Enlargement of the soft tissue of the fingertips gives a "drumstick" appearance when viewed from above		Prolonged hypoxia Emphysema Chronic obstructive pulmonary disease Advanced lung cancer
Spoon Nails (koilonychia)			
Early koilonychia	Flattening of the nail plate with an increased smoothness of the nail surface		Iron deficiency (with or without anemia) Poorly controlled diabetes (<15 yrs in duration)
Late koilonychia	Concave curvature of the nail plate		Local injury Psoriasis Chemical irritants Developmental abnormality
Beau's grooves	1-mm-wide horizontal depressions in the nail plates caused by growth arrest (involves all nails)		Acute, severe illness Prolonged febrile state Isolated periods of severe malnutrition
Pitting	Small multiple pits in the nail plate May be associated with plate thickening and onycholysis Most often involves the fingernails (several or all)		Psoriasis Alopecia areata

Pressure Ulcers[7,25]

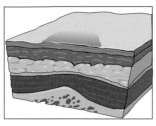
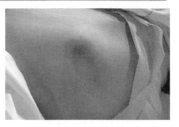

Stage I. Skin remains intact but with observable local changes in temperature (warmth or coolness), texture (firm or boggy feel), color (red in light skin; red, blue, or purple in darker skin), or sensation (pain or itching).

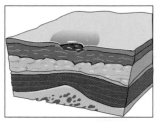
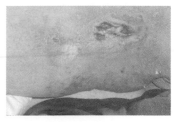

Stage II. Partial-thickness skin loss. The ulcer involves the epidermis, dermis, or both and is considered a partial-thickness skin loss. It is superficial and may look like an abrasion, blister, or shallow crater.

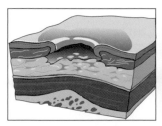
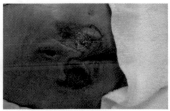

Stage III. Full-thickness skin loss. The ulcer forms a deep crater. The adjacent tissue may be involved. There is damage to or necrosis of the subcutaneous tissue, which may extend down to the underlying fascia. The fascia is not affected.

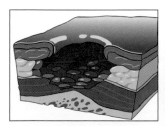
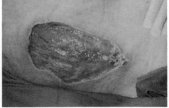

Stage IV. Full-thickness skin loss accompanied by tissue necrosis or damage to muscle, bone, or supporting structures, such as tendon or joint capsule. There is extensive tissue destruction; sinus tracts may be present.

Burn Injury Classification[25]

		CAUSE	APPEARANCE	SENSATION	COURSE
EPIDERMIS	SUPERFICIAL BURN — First-degree burn	Sunburn Ultraviolet exposure Brief exposure to flash, flame, or hot liquids	Mild to severe erythema; skin blanches with pressure; dry; no blisters; edema variable amount	Painful Hyperesthetic Tingling Pain eased by cooling	Discomfort lasts about 48 hours Desquamation in 3-7 days
DERMIS	PARTIAL-THICKNESS BURN — Second-degree burn	Superficial: Scalding liquids, semiliquids (oil, tar), or solids Deep: Immersion scald, flame	Large thick-walled blisters covering extensive area (vesiculation)	Painful	Superficial partial-thickness burn heals in 14-21 days
			Edema; mottled red base; broken epidermis; wet, shiny, weeping surface	Sensitive to cold air	Deep partial-thickness burn requires 21-28 days for healing Healing rate varies with burn depth and presence or absence of infection
SUBCUTANEOUS TISSUE	FULL-THICKNESS BURN — Third-degree or fourth-degree burn	Prolonged exposure to: Chemical, electrical, flame, scalding liquids, steam	Variable (e.g., deep red, black, white, brown) Dry surface Edema Fat exposed Tissue disrupted	Little or no pain Insensate	Full-thickness dead skin suppurates and liquefies after 2-3 weeks Spontaneous healing may be impossible but small areas may be left alone to form scarring without grafting (called secondary intent) Requires removal of eschar and subsequent split- or full-thickness skin grafting Hypertrophic scarring and wound contractures likely to develop without preventive measures

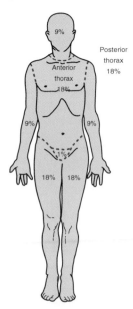

Rule of nines provides a quick method for estimating the extent of a burn injury.[25]

Pitting Edema Scale[28]

1+	Barely perceptible depression (pit)
2+	Easily identified depression (EID) (skin rebounds to its original contour within 15 sec)
3+	EID (skin rebounds to its original contour within 15–30 sec)
4+	EID (rebound >30 sec)

Signs and Symptoms of Mixed Peripheral Nerve (Lower Motor Neuron) Lesions[39]

Motor	Sensory	Sympathetic
Paralysis	Loss of or abnormal sensation	Loss of sweat glands (dryness)
Loss of reflexes		Loss of pilomotor response
Muscle wasting and atrophy	Loss of vasomotor tone: warm flushed (early); cold, white (later)	
Lost synergic action of muscles	Skin may be scaly (early); thin, smooth and shiny (later)	
Fibrosis, contractures, and adhesions	Shallower skin creases	
Joint weakness and instability	Nail changes (striations, ridges, dry, brittle, abnormal curving, luster lost)	
Decreased ROM and stiffness	Ulceration	
Disuse osteoporosis of bone		
Growth affected		

Summary of Upper Motor Neurons[37]

Tract	Origin	Function
Medial Upper Motor Neuron Tracts		
Medial corticospinal	Supplementary motor, premotor, and primary motor cerebral cortex	Control of neck, shoulder, and trunk muscles
Tectospinal	Superior colliculus of midbrain	Reflexive movement of head toward sounds or visual moving objects
Medial reticulospinal	Pontine reticular formation	Facilitates postural muscles and limb extensors
Medial vestibulospinal	Vestibular nuclei in medulla and pons	Adjusts activity in neck and upper back muscles
Lateral vestibulospinal	Vestibular nuclei in medulla and pons	Ipsilaterally facilitates LMNs to extensors; inhibits LMNs to flexors
Lateral Upper Motor Neuron Tracts		
Lateral corticospinal	Supplementary motor, premotor, and primary motor cerebral cortex	Contralateral fractionation of movement, particularly of hand movements
Rubrospinal	Red nucleus of midbrain	Facilitates contralateral upper limb flexors
Lateral reticulospinal	Medullary reticular formation	Facilitates flexor muscle motor neurons and inhibits extensor motor neurons

Tract	Origin	Function
Nonspecific Upper Motor Neuron Tracts		
Ceruleospinal	Locus ceruleus in the brain stem	Enhances the activity of interneurons and motor neurons in the spinal cord
Raphespinal	Raphe nucleus in the brain stem	Same as ceruleospinal

LMN, Lower motor neuron.

Causes of Balance Problems[7]

System	Area	Areas of Impairment	Consequences
Sensory	Peripheral	Visual system, receptors Vestibular system, receptors Somatosensory system, receptors: primarily lower extremities	Decreased ability to sense the position or movement of the head or body in relation to a static or dynamic environment
	Central	Cortical areas responsible for interpreting and integrating sensory information	Decreased ability to combine information from relevant sensory input; perception of space, true vertical or horizontal may be distorted
Motor	Peripheral	Muscles, joints, motor units	Decreased ability to execute balance strategies or reactions to postural sway
	Central	CNS areas responsible for planning, coordinating, and affecting motor control	Decreased ability to plan and coordinate postural control under static and dynamic conditions
Cognitive	Central	Cortical and limbic areas responsible for attention, arousal, and judgment	Decreased ability to remember previously successful strategies, or judge and attend to potential dangers

CNS, Central nervous system.

Normal Eye Movements[7]

Type	Description	Impairments that Increase Risk of Loss of Balance or Falls
Conjugate	Eyes move at the same time to follow object moving across visual field	Paresis/paralysis of extraocular eye muscles of one eye, diplopia
Convergence	Eyes move toward each other to follow object approaching face head-on	Paresis/paralysis of extraocular eye muscles, diplopia
Smooth pursuit	Eyes move to follow image whether head or image is moving, or both	Impaired tracking resulting from acute vestibular lesions, coordination deficits resulting from cerebellar lesions
Saccades	Quick recovery phase to resume smooth pursuit after eyes slip off an image during head or image movement, or both; function of the VOR	Slowed movement resulting from CNS disorders, such as MS or PD, or deficits, either peripheral or central
Nystagmus	Multiple slow movements of eyes interspersed rhythmically by quick recovery phases; normal if noted at ends of ranges of eye movements and after spinning (for a few seconds)	Inability to fix gaze normally, resulting from uncompensated peripheral or central vestibular deficits; vertical or oblique nystagmus may result from CNS disorders

VOR, Vestibuloocular reflex; *CNS,* central nervous system; *MS,* multiple sclerosis; *PD,* Parkinson disease.

Examples of Visual Impairments

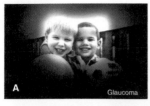

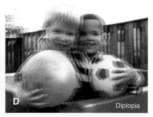

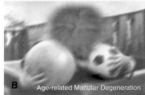

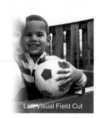

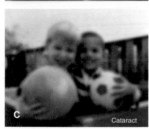

E

A, Glaucoma; **B,** macular degeneration; **C,** cataract; **D,** diplopia; **E,** left visual field cut. (Courtesy National Eye Institute, National Institutes of Health.)

Dyspnea/Angina Scale[28]

5-Grade Angina Scale		5-Grade Dyspnea Scale		10-Grade Angina/Dyspnea Scale	
0	No angina	0	No dyspnea	0	Nothing
1	Light, barely noticeable	1	Mild, noticeable	1	Very slight
2	Moderate, bothersome	2	Mild, some difficulty	2	Slight
3	Severe, very uncomfortable; preinfarction pain	3	Moderate difficulty, but can continue	3	Moderate
4	Most pain ever experienced; infarction pain	4	Severe difficulty; cannot continue	4	Somewhat severe
				5	Severe
				6	
				7	Very severe
				8	
				9	
				10	Very, very severe; maximal

Early Warning Signs of a Heart Attack[25,26]

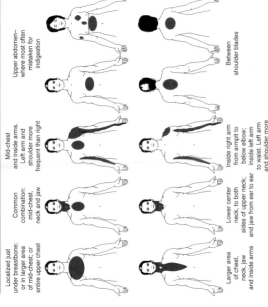

Localized just under breastbone; or in larger area of mid-chest; or entire upper chest

Common combination: mid-chest, neck and jaw

Mid-chest and inside arms. Left arm and shoulder more frequent than right

Upper abdomen—where most often mistaken for indigestion

Larger area of chest, neck, jaw and inside arms

Lower center neck; to both sides of upper neck; and jaw from ear to ear

Inside right arm from armpit to below elbow; inside left arm to waist. Left arm and shoulder more frequent than right

Between shoulder blades

Most common warning signs of heart attack

- Uncomfortable pressure, fullness, squeezing or pain in the center of the chest (prolonged)
- Pain that spreads to the throat, neck, back, jaw, shoulders, or arms
- Chest discomfort with lightheadedness, dizziness, sweating, pallor, nausea, or shortness of breath
- Prolonged symptoms unrelieved by antacids, nitroglycerin, or rest

Atypical, less common warning signs (especially women)

- Unusual chest pain (quality, location, e.g., burning, heaviness; left chest), stomach or abdominal pain
- Continuous midthoracic or interscapular pain
- Continuous neck or shoulder pain
- Isolated right biceps pain
- Pain relieved by antacids; pain unrelieved by rest or nitroglycerin
- Nausea and vomiting; flu-like manifestation without chest pain/discomfort
- Unexplained intense anxiety, weakness, or fatigue
- Breathlessness, dizziness

Multiple segmental nerve innervations shown account for varied pain patterns possible. A woman can experience any of the various patterns described but is just as likely to develop atypical symptoms of pain as depicted here.

Intervention

Manipulation Techniques[53]

Manual physical therapy approaches place an emphasis on the application of biomechanical principles in the examination and treatment of spinal disorders. Motion is analyzed with active and passive motion testing, with visualization of the spinal mechanics; the motion is best described with standardized biomechanical terminology. Passive forces are applied, with passive accessory intervertebral motion testing and mobilization/manipulation techniques, along planes of movement parallel or perpendicular to the anatomic planes of the joint surfaces. Therefore, knowledge of spinal anatomy and biomechanics is a prerequisite to learning a manual physical therapy approach for examination and treatment of the spine.

Key Terms of Manual Therapy Terminology

Accessory Motion: Those motions available in a joint that may accompany the classical movements or be passively produced when isolated from the classical movement. Accessory movements are essential to normal, full range of motion and painless function.

Component Motion: Motions that take place in a joint complex or related joint to facilitate a particular active motion.

Close-packed Position: Position of maximum congruency of a joint that is locked; statically efficient for load bearing but dynamically dangerous.

Joint Dysfunction: A state of altered mechanics; either an increase or decrease from the expected normal, or the presence of an aberrant motion.

Joint Play: Movements not under voluntary control that occur only in response to an outside force.

Kinematics: The study of the geometry of motion, independent of the kinetic influences that may be responsible for the motion. In biomechanics, the two divisions of kinematics are osteokinematics and arthrokinematics.

Loose-packed Position: Position of a joint where the capsule and ligaments are their most slack, which is unlocked; statically inefficient for load bearing, and dynamically safe.

Data from Paris SV, Loubert PV: *Foundations of clinical orthopaedics*, St. Augustine, Fla, 1990, Institute Press. (Olson MT)

Sample Manipulation Technique

LUMBOPELVIC (SACROILIAC REGION) MANIPULATION

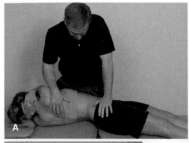
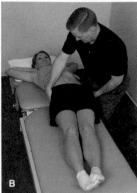
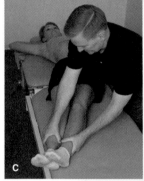
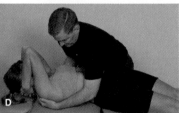
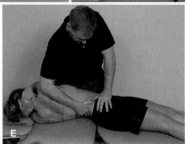

PURPOSE   This technique restores lumbopelvic mobility and reduces lumbopelvic pain.

PATIENT POSITION   The patient is supine on the treatment table.

THERAPIST POSITION   The therapist stands on the side opposite the side to be manipulated.

PROCEDURE   The pelvis is translated toward the therapist's side of the table. The therapist maximally side-bends the patient's lower extremities and trunk to the right. Without losing the right-side bending, the therapist lifts and left-rotates the trunk so that the patient rests on the left shoulder. The patient's right anterior superior iliac spine (ASIS) and ilium is contacted in a broad, comfortable manner with the therapist's left hand. The top shoulder and scapula are grasped with the therapist's right hand, and the trunk is rotated to the left, with the right-side bending maintained. Once the right ASIS starts to elevate, a counter anterior-to-posterior force is applied through the ASIS to further take up the tissue slack, and once a firm barrier to motion is reached, a high-velocity, low-amplitude thrust is performed through the pelvis in an anterior-to-posterior direction.

ALTERNATIVE TECHNIQUE   An alternative method is use of the cranial forearm and hand across the scapula and thoracic and lumbar spine to maintain the locked spinal position.

NOTES   Flynn and colleagues[a] used this technique to develop the clinical prediction rule (CPR) for manipulation for treatment of acute low back pain. This CPR was validated by Childs et al[b], who also used this technique with a different sample of patients and clinicians. This technique could be used to treat hypomobility impairments of the lower lumbar spine, lumbosacral junction, and sacroiliac joint on the targeted side.

a, Flynn T, Fritz J, Whitman J, et al: A clinical prediction rule for classifying patients with low back pain who demonstrate short-term improvement with spinal manipulation, *Spine* 27:2835–2843, 2002.

b, Childs J, Fritz J, Flynn T, et al: A clinical prediction rule to identify patients with low back pain most likely to respond to spinal manipulation: a validation study, *Ann Intern Med* 141(12):922–928, 2004.

Physical Agents[6]

Categories of Physical Agents

Category	Types	Clinical Examples
Thermal	Deep heating agents	Ultrasound, diathermy
	Superficial heating agents	Hot pack
	Cooling agents	Ice pack
Mechanical	Traction	Mechanical traction
	Compression	Elastic bandage, stockings
	Water	Whirlpool
	Sound	Ultrasound
Electromagnetic	Electromagnetic fields	Ultraviolet, laser
	Electric currents	TENS

TENS, Transcutaneous electrical nerve stimulation.

Physical Agents for Promoting Tissue Healing

Stage of Tissue Healing	Goals of Treatment	Effective Agents	Contraindicated Agents
Initial injury	Prevent further injury or bleeding	Static compression Cryotherapy	Exercise Intermittent traction Motor-level ES Thermotherapy
	Clean open wound	Hydrotherapy (immersion or nonimmersion)	
Chronic inflammation	Prevent/decrease joint stiffness	Thermotherapy Motor ES Whirlpool Fluidotherapy™	Cryotherapy
	Control pain	Thermotherapy ES Laser	
	Increase circulation	Thermotherapy ES Compression Hydrotherapy (immersion or exercise)	Cryotherapy
	Progress to proliferation stage	Pulsed ultrasound ES PSWD	
Remodeling	Regain or maintain strength	Motor ES Water exercise	Immobilization
	Regain or maintain flexibility	Thermotherapy Brief ice massage	Immobilization
	Control scar tissue formation	Compression	

ES, Electrical stimulation; *PSWD*, pulsed shortwave diathermy.

Physical Agents for the Treatment of Pain

Type of Pain	Goals of Treatment	Effective Agents	Contraindicated
Acute	Control pain	Sensory ES Cryotherapy	
	Control inflammation	Cryotherapy	Thermotherapy
	Prevent aggravation of pain	Immobilization Low-load static traction	Local exercise Motor ES
Referred	Control pain	ES Cryotherapy Thermotherapy	
Spinal radicular	Decrease nerve root inflammation	Traction	
	Decrease nerve root compression		
Pain due to malignancy	Control pain	ES Cryotherapy Superficial thermotherapy	

ES, Electrical stimulation.

Physical Agents for the Treatment of Motion Restrictions

Source of Motion Restriction	Goals of Treatment	Effective Agents	Contraindicated
Muscle weakness	Increase muscle strength	Water exercise Motor ES	Immobilization
Pain			
At rest and with motion	Control pain	ES Cryotherapy Thermotherapy PSWD Spinal traction	Exercise
With motion only	Control pain Promote tissue healing	ES Cryotherapy Thermotherapy PSWD	Exercise into pain
Soft tissue shortening	Increase tissue extensibility	Thermotherapy	Prolonged cryotherapy
	Increase tissue length	Thermotherapy or brief ice massage and stretch	
Bony block	Remove block Compensate	None Exercise Thermotherapy or brief ice massage and stretch	Stretching blocked joint

ES, Electrical stimulation; PSWD, pulsed shortwave diathermy.

Physical Agents for the Treatment of Tone Abnormalities

Tone Abnormality	Goals of Treatment	Effective Agents	Contraindicated
Hypertonicity	Decrease tone	Neutral warmth or prolonged cryotherapy to hypertonic muscles Motor ES or quick ice of antagonists	Quick ice of agonist
Hypotonicity	Increase tone	Quick ice or motor ES of agonists	Thermotherapy
Fluctuating tone	Normalize tone	Functional ES	

ES, Electrical stimulation.

Intervention and Prevention

Cardiopulmonary Drainage Postions[56]

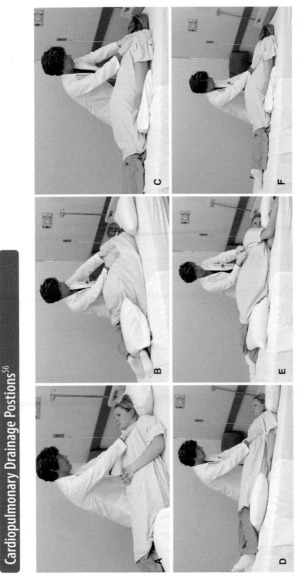

Postural drainage position for **A,** anterior segments, upper lobes; **B,** posterior segment, left upper lobe; **C,** posterior segment, right upper lobe; **D,** anterior basal segments; **E,** left lateral basal segment; and **F,** posterior basal segments.

Considerations When Selecting an Airway Clearance Technique[21]

Technique	Age of Patient	Assistant Needed	Equipment Needed	During Acute Exacerbation	Concurrent Nebulizer	Precautions	Cost
PD, percussion, vibration/shaking	Any age	Yes	Positioning aids; percussor/vibrator; devices for infants	Yes	Only in upright	May modify positions; repetitive motion injuries	Expensive if performed by caregiver long term
Manual hyperinflation	Extra care with infants	Two assistants needed	Manual ventilation bag	Yes, with tracheostomy or mechanical ventilation	Not usually	Pulmonary edema, air leak, bronchospasm, unstable, risk of pneumothorax	Expensive due to caregivers, but usually used short term
ACBT	Begin to teach at 3-4 yrs of age	Until 8-10 yrs of age	Positioning aids; percussor/vibrator	Yes	Only in upright	Only precautions for head-down positions	Cost is low if done independently
AD	Age ≥12 yrs	No	None	Best to use an alternative	No	Takes time to learn	No cost
PEP	Begin to teach at 3-4 yrs of age	Until 8-10 yrs of age	Mouthpiece or mask; PEP device; manometer	Yes	Yes, except flutter	Sinusitis, epistaxis, ear infection, risk of pneumothorax	Minimal, but devices require replacement
IPV	Adolescents and adults	While in hospital	Home unit; unit for hospital setting	May not be well tolerated	Yes	Titrate for comfort and visible chest movement	Moderate expense
HFCWO	Age ≥2-3 yrs	For young children	Air pulse generator; appropriately sized vest	Yes	Yes	Chest tube, indwelling catheter, or other device in chest area	Very expensive
Exercise	Children, adolescents, and adults	For young children	Variable	No	Medicate before exercise	Exercise-induced bronchospasm; oxygen desaturation; adjunct to ACT	Depends on type of exercise

PD, Postural drainage; *ACBT*, active cycle of breathing techniques; *AD*, autogenic drainage; *PEP*, positive expiratory pressure; *IPV*, interpulmonary percussive ventilation; *HFCWO*, high-frequency chest wall oscillation; *ACT*, airway clearance techniques.

Fall Prevention for Individuals with Increased Fall Risk[7]

Type of Patient	Examples of Intervention
Individual of advanced age	Muscle strengthening and endurance program focused on lower extremities.
	Patient education in reducing environmental hazards that represent fall risk.
Individual with a history of falls	Exercise program and gait training focused on components and types of postural control that show deficits.
	Assessment and modification of patient's environment as appropriate.
Individual with CNS pathology with chronic or progressive balance deficits	Exercise program, instruction in ADL, and gait training with assistive devices as needed.
	Patient and caregiver instruction on fall prevention and safety.

CNS, Central nervous system; *ADL*, activities of daily living.
Adapted from American Physical Therapy Association: Guide to physical therapist practice, ed 2, Alexandria, VA, 2001, APTA.

Skin Breakdown Prevention and Pressure Relief[62]

Prevention Strategy	Nursing	Physical Therapy	Occupational Therapy	Patient, Family, and Caregivers

Begin an interdisciplinary pressure relief program from day 1 of onset of SCI	• Conduct comprehensive, systematic, and consistent assessment of pressure ulcer risk factors in individuals with SCI:
	  • Assess and document on admission and reassess on a routine basis
	  • Use clinical judgment and a risk assessment tool
	  • Assess demographic, physical/medical, and psychological factors associated with pressure ulcer prevention
				Learn about the importance of comprehensive, systematic, and consistent assessment of pressure ulcer risk factors

Avoid prolonged immobilization	Implement bed turning every 2 hours	Ensure proper positioning for optimal skin protection for therapy interventions	Provide wheelchair seating and adaptive equipment for ADL	Learn about pressure relief guidelines and individualized risk factors
Areas of daily skin inspections: ischii, sacrum, coccyx, trochanters, heels, malleoli, anterior knee, shoulder, side of head, elbow, occiput, rim of ear, dorsal thoracic spine	Inspect; educate and train patient and family related to the patient's bed position, mobility status, and medical confounding factors	Educate and train patient and family about areas of inspection and use of adaptive equipment and functional activities related to inspection		Learn about methods of daily skin inspection dependent on mobility status and level of injury

Evaluate support surface	Select appropriate bed surface and monitor medical issues that may change these needs	Identify hazards of support surfaces during interventions; provide appropriate bridging for skin relief; monitor wheelchair seating and support surfaces for optimal protection	Identify hazards of support surfaces for ADLs and optimize protection and prevention; evaluate optimal seating support and monitor needs for altering these surfaces	Learn about moisture, surface shear, surface friction, and medical issues that may affect support surfaces and potential risks for skin vulnerability
Wheelchair pressure relief program	Perform and educate about weight shift in upright position every 15–30 minutes, allowing adequate oxygen replenishment to muscles	Train and educate about weight shift techniques individualized to level of injury, strength, cognitive status (power relief or manual)	Train and educate about maintenance of equipment and weight shift options (power relief or manual)	Learn about and teach caregivers the individualized skin relief schedule and methods
Mobility program training for prevention of deconditioning	Encourage patient in self-direction of care; educate about the importance of mobility to decrease the incidence of pressure ulcer development	Educate and provide individual guidelines for mobility and exercise programs for the prevention of pressure ulcer development	Educate about the importance of mobility to decrease the incidence of pressure ulcer development	Practice self-direction of care; learn about the importance of mobility in relation to decreased incidence of ulcer development
Individualized patient education program	• Consider the learning styles of patients and family • Assess understanding by questions • Clarify and give explanations, considering psychosocial issues			Ask a lot of questions

ADL, Activities of daily living.

Wheelchairs

Advantages, Disadvantages, and Possible Applications of Various Wheeled Mobility Technologies[38]

Wheeled Mobility Device	Advantages	Disadvantages	Possible Application
Semiadjustable manual wheelchair (lightweight)	Simple to use Folds for transportation Lighter weight than standard wheelchair Partial adjustability Easier to propel Durable Will accommodate custom seating	Not custom fit Lack of axle adjustability may limit manual propulsion by user Still may be too heavy for many users	Intermittent or temporary use Possible use for in-home applications if environment tolerates
Fully adjustable manual wheelchair with a folding frame (ultra-lightweight)	Very light frame Maximal adjustability, especially of rear axle position Custom fit to user Accommodates custom seating Accommodates to uneven ground by flexing Folds side to side for easy transportation	Many adjustable or removable parts More complex design, requires more maintenance Some propulsion energy lost in flex of frame	Full-time wheelchair user with permanent disability User wants to transport in trunk of vehicle Environment includes travel over uneven surfaces
Fully adjustable manual wheelchair with a rigid frame (ultra-lightweight)	Very light frame Maximal adjustability, especially of rear axle position Custom fit to user Fewer removable or adjustable parts than folding frame Accommodates custom seating	Does not accommodate to uneven terrain as easily as folding frame May be more difficult to transport in trunk of car (less compact when folded)	Full-time wheelchair user with permanent disability User wants most efficient system for propulsion Used mainly indoors or on even terrains
Power assist manual wheelchair	Light frame Maneuvers like manual wheelchair Minimizes stress on shoulders	Heavier than non-power assist More difficult to disassemble for transport	Lightweight manual wheelchair user with limited endurance or shoulder limitations Manual wheelchair user with long-distance ambulation needs or difficulty managing outdoor terrain independently

Wheeled Mobility Device	Advantages	Disadvantages	Possible Application
Tilt-in-space frame wheelchair	Allows rotation in space for pressure management or other benefits Available for both manual and powered wheelchairs	Frame often heavier and bulkier Usually does not fold for transportation If on manual wheelchair, typically has small rear wheels, requiring an attendant to propel	Wheelchair user requires rotation in space for pressure management or other medical reason, such as respiratory disease
Reclining frame wheelchair	Allows for change in seat-to-back angle, often to full supine position Available for both manual and powered wheelchairs	Frame often heavier and bulkier Rear wheels set farther back to provide larger base of support when in recline position Difficult to propel if used with manual wheelchair	Used when a need for change in seat to back angle is required Used for pressure management May be used for self-care in wheelchair May be used when supine bed transfers are required Often used when building sitting tolerance during initial rehabilitation
Powered scooter	Allows to learn powered mobility Good outdoor access Swivel seat for ease of transfers Baskets and other accessories for function, such as shopping	Only one access method Large turning radius; difficult to use in many homes Does not accommodate custom seating; few seating support options	Used with individuals who have limited endurance Often used for primarily outdoor mobility purposes
Powered wheelchair	Full access to powered mobility for both indoor and outdoor use Multiple access methods possible Accommodates custom seating supports Accommodates power seating options, such as tilt or recline	Heavy Requires van for transportation Less maneuverable than manual wheelchair Requires more initial training for optimal safety and function	Individuals who cannot propel manual wheelchair effectively Used for indoor and outdoor mobility for long distances May be used in work or school applications for part-time manual wheelchair users

Types of Manual Wheelchairs[64]

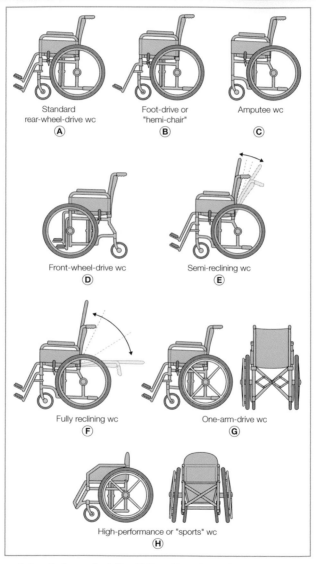

A, Standard rear-wheel-drive; **B,** Foot-drive or hemi-chair; **C,** Amputee;
D, Front-wheel drive; **E,** Semireclining; **F,** Fully reclining; **G,** One-arm drive;
H, High-performance or sports.

Types of Powered Wheelchairs[64]

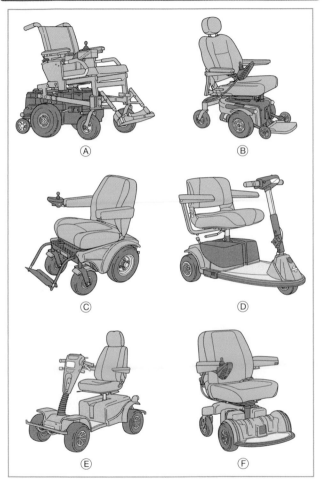

A, Direct-drive powered/rear-wheel drive; **B,** Direct-drive powered/front-wheel drive; **C,** Belt-driven powered; **D,** Three-wheeled scooter; **E,** Four-wheeled scooter; **F,** Hoveround.

Parts of a Manual Wheelchair[64]

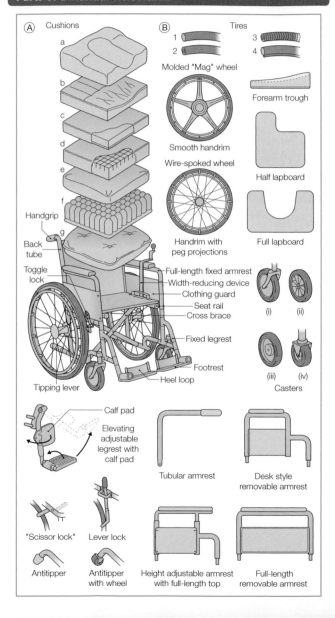

(A) Cushions
a
b
c
d
e
f
g
Handgrip
Back tube
Toggle lock
Tipping lever

(B) Tires
1
2
3
4

Molded "Mag" wheel
Smooth handrim
Wire-spoked wheel
Handrim with peg projections

Forearm trough
Half lapboard
Full lapboard

Full-length fixed armrest
Width-reducing device
Clothing guard
Seat rail
Cross brace
Fixed legrest
Footrest
Heel loop

(i)   (ii)
(iii)   (iv)
Casters

Calf pad
Elevating adjustable legrest with calf pad

"Scissor lock"   Lever lock

Antitipper   Antitipper with wheel

Tubular armrest

Desk style removable armrest

Height adjustable armrest with full-length top

Full-length removable armrest

Physical Assessment in Wheelchair Selection[62]

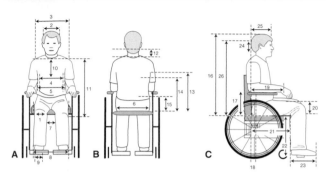

Anatomical dimensions are used to choose wheelchair and seating product dimensions.
A, Anterior view; 1 = knee width, 2 = head width, 3 = shoulder width, 4 = middle chest width, 5 = lower ribs width, 6 = seated buttock width (posterior view), 7 = interknee width, 8 = bilateral seated width, 9 = unilateral foot width, 10 = sternal height. **B,** Posterior view; 11 = seat to shoulder height (anterior view), 12 = cervical length, 13 = seat to axilla height, 14 = seat to inferior angle of the scapula, 15 = seat to posterior ilium. **C,** Lateral view; 16 = seat to top of head, 17 = seat to elbow height, 18 = vertical orientation from floor past posterior occiput, 19 = forearm length, 20 = thigh or lap height from seat, 21 = axle to posterior leg, 22 = footrest to seat height, 23 = foot length, 24 = posterior occiput to superior cervical height, 25 = head length.

TYPE

A, Pressure-relief seat cushions; a. Contoured foam, b. Contoured foam base with gel-filled pad, c. Viscoelastic foam with casing, d. Polyurethane foam, e. Gel enclosed in a nonbreathing plastic casing, f. Air-filled villous ROHO cushion, g. Water-filled seat; **B,** Tires, 1. Solid hard rubber tires, 2. Pneumatic inner tube, 3. Semipneumatic tire with coil-reinforced zero pressure tire (ZPT) inner tube, 4. Semipneumatic tire with solid foam ZPT inner tube; Casters: i. Standard 8-inch diameter with solid rubber tire, ii. 8-inch diameter with semipneumatic tire, iii. 8-inch diameter with pneumatic tire, iv. 5-inch diameter with solid rubber tire (ROHO cushion is a product of ROHO Inc., Belleville, IL.)

For figure see page 174

Manual Mobility *versus* Powered Mobility Considerations[52]

Consideration	Manual Mobility Questions	Powered Mobility Questions
Function	Is the person able to propel a manual w/c using upper and/or lower extremities at household and community distances? Has the person been given an opportunity to use technology that would maximize potential to propel a manual w/c (e.g., an adjustable w/c that has been set up appropriately for the person)?	Is the person's strength or endurance such that manual w/c propulsion is not possible? Does the typical daily routine require propulsion beyond the limits of the individual's endurance or place the person at high risk for orthopedic problems? Will use of a manual w/c result in secondary complications (i.e., pelvic obliquity or scoliosis)?
Transportation	What kind of transportation is available for a manual w/c? Will the person load the w/c independently? What w/c frame and components will improve independence?	Does the person have access to transportation (personal or public) for powered mobility? Are tie downs and a lift device available and appropriate for powered mobility? Is obtaining powered and manual mobility feasible for the person?
Environment	Will the person primarily use the w/c inside the home? Is the user able to self-propel in the community or rely on assistance? What is the terrain like in the community (e.g., hilly, flat, rocky, etc.)?	Is powered mobility necessary for independence because of the distances traveled or difficult terrain?
Cognition	Is the person able to safely propel a manual w/c? Because of poor judgment or safety concerns, does the clinician need to restrict accessibility?	Does the person understand cause and effect? Does the person exhibit cognitive impairments in memory, problem solving, or impulse control that may prohibit the use of a power w/c? Is the intended user only safe in familiar environments?
Vocational	Can the person manage daily routines including work and school activities using a manual w/c?	Is powered mobility necessary for the person to efficiently manage work and school activities without being exhausted?
Medical complications	What medical complications are present that would inhibit the person's ability to use a manual w/c?	Does the person have cardiopulmonary problems? Is the person unable to sustain functional cardiac output to push a manual w/c household distances?

w/c, Wheelchair.

Seating Systems[22]

Seating Component	Indications for Use	Postural and Functional Considerations
Solid insert	Insert can provide a level base of support on the sling wheelchair seat. Slide insert inside the cover and under the cushion, and secure to cushion base with Velcro. The cushion cover usually has Velcro to attach the cushion securely to sling upholstery of the wheelchair.	A sling wheelchair seat encourages a posterior pelvic tilt with hip adduction and internal rotation. This sets an individual up for a "slumped" posture. A solid insert is essential to provide a firm and level base of support on the sling wheelchair seat. This facilitates more neutral pelvic positioning for upright posture and upper body movement for functional activities.
1.5-inch seat wedge	Wedge slides inside the cushion cover, under the cushion. Wedge can provide an anterior or posterior seat tilt.	Wedge is a lightweight, easy-to-remove component to use for an anterior-sloped seat or a posterior-sloped seat. An anterior tilt would facilitate upright positioning for an individual who is working at a workstation or propelling with one arm and one foot. A posterior tilt can assist with decreasing extensor spasticity or creating a set, slight tilt for increased postural support in a standard wheelchair.
Solid seat 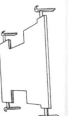	Remove wheelchair upholstery to install. To mount, solid seat hooks lock down on seat rails of wheelchair. The adjustable hooks can be positioned to provide an anterior or posterior tilt of solid seat and cushion on wheelchair frame.	Seat also encourages neutral pelvic alignment and lower extremity alignment. One concern is that it adds a significant amount of weight to the wheelchair. Unless necessary to achieve a low seat-to-floor height that cannot be achieved with a super-low wheelchair, the weight disadvantage outweighs the positioning advantages.
Foam cushion 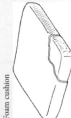	Foam linear cushions provide a stable base of support for individuals with mild postural support needs. The foam comes in varying densities and can be layered in different densities to provide support, comfort, and some pressure relief.	Cushions can enhance sitting posture and pressure distribution, and increase comfort.

Continued

Seating Component	Indications for Use	Postural and Functional Considerations
Pressure-relieving cushion (fluid medium) 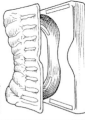	A firm, contoured cushion base with pressure-relieving gel fluid pad on top provides stability and a high level of pressure relief appropriate for all individuals who need moderate to significant postural support and pressure relief. The gel bladder allows the pelvis to sink into it for full contact support for adequate pressure distribution to minimize the risk of pressure sores.	These off-the-shelf cushions provide a superior level of pressure relief and good pelvic stability. This stability is important for improved balance and for adequate support. It can improve function at a wheelchair level and minimize compensatory posturing.
Pressure-relieving cushion (air medium) 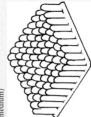	The air medium allows the seated individual to sink into this cushion for contoured support and a high degree of pressure distribution to minimize the risk of pressure sores.	The pressure relief and lightweight qualities of this cushion are unsurpassed. However, this cushion does not provide any stability, and additional postural supports such as hip guides and adductors are essential for optimal alignment. These supports increase weight of the whole wheelchair system. Another concern is the ongoing maintenance required with this cushion.
Contoured foam cushion 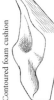	Contoured foam cushion provides an increased surface area of support and pressure relief for individuals with mild to moderate support and pressure relief needs. A variety of foam densities are available.	The combination of stability and pressure relief is a major advantage to this cushion. The weight is a consideration; however, the advantage of a stable and pressure-relieving base of support minimizes the need for external supports.

Lumbar-sacral back support	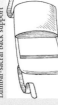	This component can provide support to the lumbar-sacral region to support the pelvis in neutral pelvic alignment. A more secure attachment method is recommended to keep it in position.	This support is a low-cost method to provide minimal postural support for increased spinal-pelvic alignment. The support is easy to remove, which is an advantage for car transport, but a disadvantage because the support is not stable and can shift out of place easily.
Solid back support	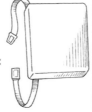	The solid back insert provides firm support to facilitate improved postural alignment for individuals with good pelvic and trunk control. The support is easy to remove for transportability of the wheelchair and usually is attached to the wheelchair back canes with Velcro straps.	This support is a low-cost method to provide minimal postural support for increased spinal-pelvic alignment. The support is easy to remove, which is an advantage for car transport, but a disadvantage because the support is not stable and can shift out of place easily.
Pita back	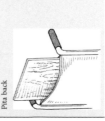	This solid back insert provides a firm support to facilitate improved postural alignment for individuals with good pelvic and trunk control. The support is easy to remove for transportability of the wheelchair and slides into and out of a pocket in the back support upholstery.	This simple, low-cost back support can provide minimal postural support for increased spinal-pelvic alignment. The lack of foam makes the support easy to use; however, lack of sufficient padding is a concern for individuals using the wheelchair as a primary means of mobility.

Continued

Seating Component	Indications for Use	Postural and Functional Considerations
Linear back support	This solid back insert provides a more durable back support for increased spinal-pelvic alignment, is beneficial for individuals with good postural control, is attached to the wheelchair frame with quick-release hardware, and usually is linear with a solid posterior base with foam in front. The support may be covered in vinyl or other materials.	This is a planar back support to enhance upright sitting. The adjustable mounting brackets make it possible to open up seat-to-back angle to accommodate a hip range of motion limitation or for increased postural support and balance via gravity. This hardware is durable. One concern is the weight added to the wheelchair.
Adjustable-angle off-the-shelf back support	This back support can be attached to the wheelchair with quick-release hardware. The support has generic, gentle contours that provide a guide for increased postural alignment for individuals with mild to moderate positioning needs and can be used in its original configuration or can accommodate a contoured foam in-place back support.	This back support provides mild contour to facilitate neutral trunk posturing and increased spinal-pelvic alignment. The angle can be adjusted to open up seat-to-back angle to accommodate a hip range of motion limitation or for increased postural support and balance via gravity. This support is a lightweight option that provides good support. One concern is that more durable hardware may be necessary for individuals with significant spasticity.
Adjustable-angle custom back support	This rigid back support can be attached to the wheelchair with quick-release or stationary hardware. The support often is positioned at an angle with a custom-contoured amount of support. The shell can be reused if the foam insert needs to be modified. This support benefits individuals with moderate to significant trunk weaknesses and/or flexible or fixed postural deformities.	This back support can provide moderate to significant support for individuals with flexible and fixed deformities. The hardware can open up the seat-to-back angle for the foregoing reasons. The contoured support provides maximum surface area contact to maximize alignment, accommodate deformities, and maximize pressure distribution to minimize the risk for increased deformities and pressure sores.

Pelvic positioning support	Pelvic supports are designed to maintain optimal pelvic alignment and minimize an individual's risk for sliding out of the wheelchair. They are mounted to the seat frame via screws or straps and are available with various angles of pull and various buckles such as auto and airline style.	This support can be positioned at various angles depending on the individual's needs and functional level. A pelvic belt at the traditional 45 degrees can limit pelvic mobility for an anterior weight shift for forward reach and functioning at a table. Padded belts are available to minimize pressure concerns, and various buckles are available for maximum independence with opening/closing.
Leg adductors	The adductor can be attached to the wheelchair cushion base, under the seat, or on the footrest hanger, and is designed to maximize lower extremity alignment and prevent the legs from rolling into abduction or external hip rotation.	Adductors can facilitate increased lower extremity alignment to minimize an individual's risk of increased deformity and pain. The size of the adductor can limit side-to-side transfers; a removable one can provide adequate support and increased safety with side transfers.
Hip guides	Hip guides provide support to maximize pelvic alignment, can be contoured or linear, and usually are made of different density foams, with a solid back. Hip guides can be mounted onto the wheelchair armrests, seat pan, or back canes. The hardware can be fixed or removable. 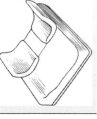	Hip guides can provide a third point of control for individuals with fixed or flexible spinal curves or individuals who have a pelvic obliquity. Removable hardware is necessary for individuals who perform side-to-side transfers.

Continued

Seating Component	Indications for Use	Postural and Functional Considerations
Medial knee block (pommel) with flip-down hardware 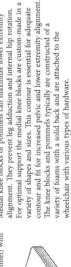	Medial knee blocks or pommels can maximize lower extremity alignment. They prevent leg adduction and internal hip rotation. For optimal support the medial knee blocks are custom-made in a variety of shapes and sizes. This contour is essential for adequate contour and fit for increased pelvic and lower extremity alignment. The knee blocks and pommels typically are constructed of a variety of foams with a solid back and are attached to the wheelchair with various types of hardware.	Medial knee blocks are often necessary for individuals with severe spasticity. They are most successful when used with the other postural supports to maximize overall postural alignment. They can promote increased lower extremity alignment. Small pommels are helpful as a guide for more neutral lower extremity posturing.
Pelvic obliquity build-up	This component usually is mounted under the gel pad or created with foams; it can be a gel or foam medium and can provide increased support under the weaker side to accommodate for muscle atrophy, as well as level out the pelvis for improved pelvic alignment, to provide a more level foundation from which the body can function. This component may be used with a hip guide to minimize lateral tilting of the pelvis for increased spinal-pelvic alignment. It also may be used under the higher side to support a fixed pelvic obliquity adequately and minimize the risk of increased deformity.	Foam or gel inserts are helpful for individuals with asymmetrical muscle strength. They can compensate for the decreased muscle bulk to facilitate a more level pelvic position. When used with hip guides, inserts can support optimal pelvic alignment in individuals who have a flexible pelvis. One concern is the amount of pressure the inserts place on the ipsilateral ischial tuberosity. Monitoring of pressure with this treatment approach is important.

Lateral trunk supports, straight and curved

These supports usually are mounted off the back support or back canes and are available in various sizes in planar or contoured levels of support. The hardware to mount to the wheelchair can be stationary or quick release, which is beneficial for individuals with trunk weakness or a tendency to lean to one side. Another point of control, usually via hip guides, is necessary for adequate trunk support to correct a flexible deformity or accommodate a fixed deformity.

Individuals who have decreased trunk support often hold themselves upright with their upper extremities. Lateral supports can provide increased trunk support to these individuals so that they can use their extremities for bilateral upper extremity tasks. Lateral supports also can provide the upper two points of control to correct or accommodate a lateral spinal curve for increased midline positioning in the wheelchair. The swing-away hardware is helpful with providing adequate support and shifting out of the way for transfers, dressing, and overall positioning in the wheelchair. Lateral support hardware that aggressively contours to the back support is necessary to get the hardware out of the way for adequate upper extremity mobility. Curved lateral support pads provide improved contour and support over planar lateral support pads.

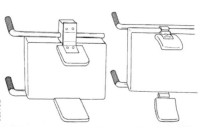

Continued

Seating Component	Indications for Use	Postural and Functional Considerations
Harness/anterior chest support	Anterior chest supports can be mounted to the wheelchair via the back support of back canes and seat rails. They are available in a variety of styles and are beneficial for individuals with severe trunk weakness. These supports often are used with a tilt or recline seating system to maximize postural support when more upright against gravity.	This component can provide anterior trunk support to allow an individual with poor trunk control to be more upright against gravity, which is helpful for more dynamic, engaging activities (i.e., working at a desk). Therapists should consider this component after evaluating a recline or tilt-in-space seating system for increased postural support in a more sedentary, posterior position. The component is helpful for maximum trunk support for increased safety and stability when negotiating varying terrain (i.e., ramps and door saddles).
Head/neck support	Head/neck supports can be mounted to the back support via quick-release hardware. They are essential to provide adequate head support for individuals with poor head or neck control.	This component is necessary for individuals with fair head control and for head and neck support when an individual tilts back for pressure relief or improved postural support. Additional pads and headbands are available for individuals with significant head positioning needs. This should be adjusted to support the head in neutral alignment for optimal functioning (i.e., respiration and feeding) and speech.

Wheel lock extension	Wheel lock extensions can be mounted over the existing wheel lock handle. They are available in various sizes. They provide a longer lever arm to make it possible to access and lock/unlock the wheel locks if an individual cannot negotiate the standard wheel lock.	Extensions are important for maximum independence and to stabilize the wheelchair for functioning and safety with transfers to and from the wheelchair.
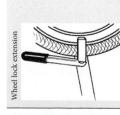		
Upper extremity support, full and half lap trays	Lap trays can be mounted over the arm pad with "slide" hardware, with an additional strap for stability, if necessary. They come in full or half tray models in various sizes. They can provide individuals with a support surface for their paretic upper extremity.	Adequate upper extremity support is essential to minimize an individual's risk for increased shoulder pain and deformity. A lap tray can provide a work surface for functional activities such as writing and feeding. The clear version can provide the individual with a clear view of the feet for maximum safety with wheelchair propulsion. Upper extremity edema is often present in individuals who are unable to move their upper extremity functionally. A lap tray can facilitate increased awareness of this extremity for edema management and positioning of the upper extremity to decrease the edema.
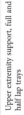 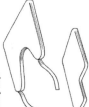		
Arm trough	An arm trough can be mounted on the standard armrest in place of the arm pad. The trough can provide more aggressive support for adequate upper extremity joint protection.	An arm trough provides optimal support for individuals with decreased upper extremity control, which is important to minimize the risk for pain, subluxation, and edema. An arm trough can provide an individual with a surface for upper extremity weight bearing for functional reaching activities or for repositioning the body in the wheelchair.

Various Types of Seating Fabrication Materials[51]

Cushion Type	Advantages	Disadvantages
Foam	Inexpensive Lightweight Nothing leaks	Affected by light and air, which cause degradation of the foam Loses shape
Gel/viscous fluid	Good pressure relief Easier than air to maintain	Heavy Chance of leakage May bottom out
Air without foam	Lightweight Waterproof Good pressure distribution over entire seated surface Adjustable via valves to relieve sores or provide postural support	Less stable Chance of puncture/damage High maintenance
Thermoplastic elastomer/urethane honeycomb	Lightweight Good support No risk of leakage Machine washable/dryable	Can produce unwanted shear force if used without a cover
Custom-molded cushions	Designed to meet individual pressure and positioning needs	Expensive No ability to modify once fabricated

Major Wheelchair Manufacturers[14]

Manufacturer	Types of Wheelchairs	Web Address
Alber (in the USA) Frank Mobility Systems, Inc. 888-426-8581	Stair-climbing wheelchair; add-on power unit	http://www.ulrich-alber.de/en/index.php
Altimate Medical, Inc. 800-342-8968	Standing systems	http://www.easystand.com
Amigo Mobility International, Inc. 800-692-6446	Scooters	http://www.myamigo.com
Bruno Independent Living Aids 800-882-8183	Adult and pediatric scooters, sedan and van wheelchair lifts	http://www.bruno.com
Columbia Medical 562-282-0244	Dependent mobility bases	http://www.columbiamedical.com
Convaid, Inc.	Dependent mobility bases, transport chairs	http://www.convaid.com
ConvaQuip	Bariatric wheelchairs	http://www.convaquip.com
Etac (in the USA) Balder USA, Inc. 888-422-5337	Independent manual wheelchairs for children and adults	http://www.etac.com

Manufacturer	Types of Wheelchairs	Web Address
Graham-Field Health Products	Dependent and independent manual and powered wheelchairs, sports wheelchairs, adult and pediatric chairs, tilt chairs	http://www.grahamfield.com/
Freedom Designs 800-331-8551	Pediatric wheelchairs, tilt in space wheelchairs	http://www.freedomdesigns.com
Gendron, Inc. 800-537-2521	Bariatric manual and power wheelchairs	http://www.gendroninc.com
Innovative Products, Inc. 800-950-5185	Pediatric powered mobility	http://www.mobility4kids.com
Invacare 800-333-6900	Manual, power, and sports wheelchairs	http://www.invacare.com
Levo USA, Inc. 888-538-6872	Manual and powered stand-up wheelchairs for adults and children	http://www.levousa.net
Life Stand (Vivre-Debout) (In the USA) Frank Mobility Systems, Inc. 888-426-8581	Manual and powered stand-up wheelchairs for adults and children	http://www.lifestand-usa.com
Mulholland Positioning Systems, Inc. 800-543-4769	A variety of standing systems, pediatric wheeled bases and tilt bases	http://www.mulhollandinc.com
Otto Bock 800-328-4058	Pediatric seating and positioning, adult positioning, manual and power wheelchairs	http://www.ottobockus.com
PDG 888-858-4422	Wheelchairs for individuals with special needs, such as bariatric chairs, high agitation, and manual tilt wheelchairs	http://www.pdgmobility.com
Permobil, Inc. 800-736-0925	Stand-up powered wheelchairs; powered wheelchairs with elevating seats; sports wheelchairs, lightweight manual wheelchairs	http://www.permobil.com
Pride Mobility Products Corp. USA 800-800-8586 Canada 888-570-1113	Manual and electrically powered wheelchairs, scooters	http://www.pridemobility.com
Snug Seat 800-336-7684	Specialty bases for children and adults, car seats, dependent and independent mobility bases, pediatric wheelchairs	http://www.snugseat.com

Continued

Manufacturer	Types of Wheelchairs	Web Address
Sunrise Medical 800-333-4000	Dependent and independent manual bases, sports wheelchairs, lightweight manual wheelchairs, powered wheelchairs, add-on power unit; adult and pediatric wheelchairs, tilt wheelchairs and scooters	http://www.sunrisemedical.com
TiLite 800-545-2266	Adult and pediatric titanium wheelchairs; manual wheelchair; sports wheelchair; ASK—see power	http://www.tilite.com http://www.titaniumsports.com

Assistive Devices for Activities of Daily Living

Dressing
- Larger buttons or zippers with a pull tab
- Velcro
- Elastic waist pants
- Front-opening garments

Eating/Meal Preparation
- Built-up handles on eating utensils
- Weighted utensils or cuff weight on the wrist
- Plate guard or scoop dish
- Straws to drink from glasses
- Utility carts to prevent lifting objects
- Stabilizing pads under the bowls when mixing
- Electric can openers
- Pots/pans with two handles
- Crock pots and microwaves
- Prepared foods such as prewashed/cut salads
- Carts to transfer items from the work area, to the table, to the sink, and to the refrigerator

Personal Hygiene
- Long handles on a comb, brush, other
- Electric toothbrushes

Environmental
- Lever-type door handles
- Large button phones
- Enlarged pen or pencils

Other/Safety
- Blunt scissors
- Eliminate ironing
- Dust mitts when dusting
- Eliminate objects from the home that could be broken easily such as knick-knacks

Home Exercise Examples[44]

Suggested Postsurgical Home Maintenance after Total Shoulder Arthroplasty

These are general guidelines; however, specific guidance and details need to be addressed by the physical therapist. Consideration must be given according to the status and capabilities of the patient.

Early phase: 0–6 weeks

GOALS FOR THE PERIOD: Aware of sleeping positions, independent with home exercise program, control pain, maintain range of motion (ROM) of proximal and distal joints, protect healing structures

Exercises:

1. Instruct the patient on sleeping positions and encourage experimentation (usually semireclined with upper extremities [UE] supported by pillows or bolster).
2. When appropriate, initiate passive range of motion (PROM) or self-assisted ROM at the shoulder (avoid external rotation [ER] beyond 40°).
3. Wear a sling for comfort.
4. Have the patient perform active range of motion (AROM) of the wrist and hand, elbow flexion only with humerus supported to decrease strain on biceps tendon, and AROM of cervical spine and thoracic spine through the cardinal planes.

Midphases: 6–12 weeks

GOALS FOR THE PERIOD: Increase shoulder ROM, initiate strengthening, increase functional activities

Exercises:

1. Continue previously mentioned ROM exercises.
2. Initiate submaximal isometrics (being careful not to irritate the healing subscapularis muscle).
3. Perform active assistive range of motion (A/AROM) exercises in supine, then progress to AROM in supine, and finally AROM in sitting as able (the patient must perform exercises correctly).

Late phases: 13 weeks to discharge

GOALS FOR THE PERIOD: Return to activities (including overhead activities), increase ROM, improve strength, improve neuromuscular control

Exercises:

1. Continue with previously mentioned exercises as needed.
2. Use AROM for concentric and eccentric strengthening at the shoulder.
3. Perform rotator cuff strengthening (elevation exercises must be performed correctly).

Suggested Postsurgical Home Maintenance after Anterior Cruciate Ligament Reconstruction

Home exercises are progressed through the four phases of rehabilitation based on the patient's tolerance to activity. Any increase in edema, pain, or laxity should be addressed early, and exercises should be modified to eliminate complications.

Weeks 1–4

GOALS FOR THE PERIOD: Manage pain and edema, improve quadriceps/hamstring contractions, improve ROM

Pain and Edema

1. Cryotherapy with elevation 20–30 minutes with ankle pumps (10 repetitions every minute)
2. Use of home ES unit

Strength

1. Isometrics: quadriceps and hamstring sets isolation and contractions, 10–30 repetitions (can also be done with elevation)

ROM Exercises

1. Supine knee extension
2. Prone heel hangs
3. Heel slides
4. Supine wall slides (supine with involved foot against the wall, gravity assisted into flexion)

AROM Exercises (brace locked):

1. Hip: flexion, extension, abduction, adduction, abduction with external rotation (ER)
2. Standing hamstring curls

Gait Training

1. Gait training using crutches: weight bearing as tolerated, weaning as appropriate
2. Use small obstacles to work on swing phase of gait, clearing involved leg (hip flexion, knee flexion, and ankle dorsiflexion)
3. Once full weight bearing obtained, work on single-limb balance activities
(Perform exercises three times a day with repetitions and sets determined by strength—usually two sets of as many as 30 repetitions.)

Weeks 5–8

GOALS FOR THE PERIOD: Progress ROM, increase functional strength of hip, knee, and ankle

ROM Exercises

1. Continue PROM exercises on an as-needed basis (ROM as needed, progress to prescribed duration with weight on top of knee if full extension is not reached at this time).
2. Add seated passive flexion.

Strength

1. Add step up and down with appropriate-height object (local phone book versus county phone book) and single-limb balance activities.
2. Follow a walking program (as much as 45 minutes of continuous walking on level surfaces daily).
3. Progress back into therapy or community gym environment for cardiovascular exercises: bike, elliptical, treadmill (forward and reverse). Progress upper extremity exercise program to weight-bearing–position gym activities (progressed to include cardiovascular, proprioceptive, and neuromuscular training techniques).

Gait Training

1. Work on single-limb balance and walking figure-eight and box patterns.
2. Try walking box and figure-eight patterns.

Weeks 9–16

GOALS FOR THE PERIOD: Progress functional activities, prepare to return to sport or activity

ROM Exercises

1. Should be close to full ROM by this time. Maintenance program should be initiated.

Strength

1. Periodize gym program; initiate running program when appropriate (usually about 3 months).
2. Progress neuromuscular (balance and coordination) training, emphasizing proper LE alignment with activities.
3. Progress balance and coordination activities and continue education on injury prevention with return to specific sport or activity.
4. Add one-legged hopping and jumping activities once cleared for running (usually about week 12).
5. Begin foundational exercises for return to sport, emphasizing LE control and neuromuscular training principles.

Week 17 and Beyond

GOALS FOR THE PERIOD: Progress back to sport or activity

ROM Exercises:

1. Maintenance

Strength:

1. Gym-based workouts continuing to emphasize proprioceptive and neuromuscular training techniques
2. Perform exercises specific to sport
3. Reassess and progress the periodization program for athlete to adequately prepare for return to sport

Phases of Rehabilitation

Sample of the Phases for Carpal Tunnel Release Postsurgical Rehabilitation

Rehabilitation Phase	Criteria to Progress to this Phase	Anticipated Impairments and Functional Limitations	Intervention	Goal	Rationale
Phase Ia Postoperative 1–10 days	Postoperative	• Edema • Pain • Limited ROM of UE • Limited functional use of UE	• Instruct on surgical site protection and monitor for drainage • Elevate and ice hand and wrist • AROM: Shoulder—all ranges Elbow—all ranges Forearm—pronation, supination Fingers—tendon gliding thumb AROM all ranges	• Prevent infection and postoperative complications • Manage edema • Decrease pain • Full AROM of shoulder, elbow, forearm • Increase AROM of fingers within limits of postoperative dressing	• Catch infection early to prevent further complications • Begin to have patient self-manage edema and pain • Restore ROM to prepare UE for functional use • Limit scar adhesions to tendons and nerves
Phase Ib Postoperative 11–21 days	No signs of infection Sutures removed	• Edema • Pain • Limited functional use of UE • Limited AROM of hand and wrist • Limited strength of hand and wrist	• Hot pack • ES • Ultrasound, phonophoresis • Iontophoresis • Cryotherapy • Retrograde massage • Isometrics: Wrist—flexion, extension	• Decrease postoperative pain by 50% • Manage edema • Increase strength and facilitate gross grasp and wrist stabilization • Full AROM of shoulder, elbow, and forearm	• Modalities to manage edema and decrease pain; help in preparation for stretching and strengthening • Massage to facilitate lymphatic return • Increased wrist stabilization strength

- Scar sensitivity, adhesions, and thickening
- Persistent paresthesia, especially at night
- Limited hand function
- Limited patient knowledge of neutral wrist positioning

- AROM: Progress exercises as indicated and add wrist—extension, radial deviation, and ulnar deviation
- AROM: Progressive resistance exercises (PREs)—Paper crunches, rice gripping
- Wrist splint worn at night as needed
- Scar desensitization: gentle manual massage, mini-vibrator massage, add different textures
- Mobilization of the median nerve

Instruct patient in the following:
- Proper use of hand protection while performing self-care
- Neutral wrist positioning
- Nerve gliding techniques
- Fabricate scar conformer

- AROM of Wrist: Extension 45° Radial deviation 20° Ulnar deviation 30° Thumb—Opposition to tip of small finger Finger—Flexion to 1 cm of distal palmar crease
- Decrease sensitivity of scar
- Increase mobility of scar
- Decrease scar adhesion to flexor tendons, skin, and median nerve
- Decrease paresthesia
- Promote independent self-care
- Maintain neutral wrist position during exercises
- Encourage self-management of exercise program
- Fatten and or soften scar

- Promote full return of UE AROM, continuation of tendon gliding exercises to decrease scar adhesion
- Wrist flexion exercises are contraindicated until 21 days after surgery to prevent bowstringing of tendons
- Strengthening and improvement of endurance of wrist and hand while maintaining neutral position
- Encouragement of wrist extension with finger flexion
- Neutral position to minimize pressure on median nerve
- Organized sensory input normalizes sensory interpretation
- Early motion organizes collagen development in scar and limits scar from restricting median nerve
- Initiation of self-management
- Minimizing of development of pillar pain
- Incorporation of neutral position during exercises and ADLs to prevent complications
- Pressure applied over a scar organizes collagen

Continued

Rehabilitation Phase	Criteria to Progress to this Phase	Anticipated Impairments and Functional Limitations	Intervention	Goal	Rationale
Phase II Postoperative 4-6 weeks	• Pain controlled • No loss of ROM • No loss of strength • Well-healed incision	• Mild edema • Mild pain • Limited AROM of wrist, fingers, and thumb • Scar sensitivity • Scar adhesion • Scar raised or thickened • Limited UE strength • Limited ability to perform light ADL involving gripping and twisting • Limited knowledge of proper work environment organization (ergonomics) • Limited tolerance to repetitive finger and hand use	• Continuation of modalities as indicated from Phase Ib • Continuation of the following: • Scar desensitization techniques • Retrograde massage • AROM and PREs • Scar conformer at night • Progress firmness of manual scar massage and use large vibrator to massage scar Add the following: • PROM (stretches): Pectoralis Composite motions of the following: 1. Wrist flexion, forearm pronation, and elbow extension 2. Wrist extension, forearm pronation, and elbow extension 3. Wrist extension, forearm supination, and elbow extension • AROM: Wrist flexion • Putty exercises (light resistive putty) • Finger pinch • Finger grip • Isotonics:	• Resolve edema in fingers • Decrease pain by 70% • Decrease sensitivity of scar and increase scar mobility • Decrease scar adhesion to flexor tendon, skin, and median nerve • Increase tolerance of UE to reaching away from body • AROM of wrist: Extension 60° Radial deviation 25° Ulnar deviation 35° • Make a full fist to DPC • Thumb to DPC at base of small finger • Grip strength 30%-50% of uninvolved hand • Wrist strength 80%-90% • Proximal strength greater than 85%	• Decrease reliance on modalities and increase patient's ability to self-manage edema and pain • Continuation of exercises as indicated to allow progression of program as tolerated by patient response to treatment • Scar should now be able to handle increased mobilization techniques • UE stretches to elongate muscle tendon units for increased function • Healing of transverse carpal tunnel ligament is adequate to prevent bowstringing of the flexor tendons • Monitor triggering of one or more digits, stop gripping exercises, and treat per physician's orders • Upper quarter strengthening as a functional unit • Initiate exercises with low repetitions to prevent development of tenosynovitis and pillar pain

Phase		Interventions	Goals
		• Upper quarter exercises as in Table 5-3 (using 1- or 2-lb weights) Wrist (weight well)—Flexion, extension (begin with 0–2 lb and progress as indicated) Forearm—Pronation supination (progress as indicated) • Patient education regarding body mechanics, joint protection, and modification of ADL using adaptive equipment (grip-assistive devices) • Ergonomic evaluation • Work-simulated exercises, emphasizing neutral position of the wrists and pacing tasks; may need handwriting retraining	• Lift and carry 3–5 lb with involved hand • Independence with ADL using assistive devices as necessary and limiting exposure to heavy grasping activities • Organize work environment to decrease potential for reinjury and maximize efficiency • Work simulation for 10 minutes, alternating tasks	• Use appropriate assistive device to prevent reinjury and increase independence with ADL; avoiding heavier gripping activities such as vacuuming, laundry, and yard work; use forearms to carry versus finger grip (groceries in paper bags versus plastic) • Promote self-management of symptoms and prevent reinjury in the work environment • Prepare for return to work
Phase III Postoperative 6–12 weeks	Patients need to perform job that requires heavy lifting	• Limited UE and grip strength • Limited UE and grip endurance	• Continuation of exercises and stretches in Phases I and II as indicated • Progress UE strengthening exercises, emphasizing endurance for return to work activities • Functional capacity evaluation • Work-simulated activities	• Decrease number of exercises and stretches • Adequate strength to return to work activities full time • Self-management of symptoms	• Increase efficiency of home exercises in self-management of condition • Promote muscle balance of UE • Assess potential to return to work • Initiate appropriate program (work hardening, work conditioning, or supervised gym program)

Sample Form to Track Milestones after Total Knee Arthroplasty[11]

HSS TOTAL KNEE ARTHROPLASTY-FUNCTIONAL MILESTONES FORM

REHABILITATION DEPARTMENT
PT Initials: _____
Diagnosis: _____ Age: _____
Right/Left/Bilateral　Initial/Revision
Unicondylar ☐
WBAT　PWB　TTWB　NWB
Height _____(in) Weight _____(lbs)　**Day of Surgery:** Su M T W Th F Sa

Anesthesia:　EPI　GEN
PCA:　EPI　IV
Femoral Nerve Block:　YES　NO

Pre-op class:　YES　NO
Pre-op Amb: w/c bound　<1　1–5　6–10　>10 Blocks
Pre-op Assistive Device: Cane/Crutches/Walker/None
Need to negotiate stairs:　YES　NO
Pre-op Lives Alone:　YES　NO

	RR	1	2	3	4	5	6	7	8	9	10	11	12	13	14	15
BID																
Discharge																
Stairs Unassisted																
Stairs Aassisted																
Cane Unassisted																
Cane Aassisted																
Walker Unassisted																
Walker Aassisted																
Stand Only																
Transfer Unassisted																
Transfer Assisted																
Dangle Unassisted																
Dangle Assisted																
CPM																
Active Ext R																
Active Flex R																
Active Ext L																
Active Flex L																
Pain Level																
Date of Surgery																
P.O.D.	RR	1	2	3	4	5	6	7	8	9	10	11	12	13	14	15

Discharge To:　　Home　　　　　　　　　　Rehab　　　　　SNF
If D/c to home:　　Home PT　　　　　　　　Outpatient　　No PT
If D/c to home, with:　Family/Friends/Other　Alone

Complications/PT Held: _____
_____
_____
_____

Sample Form to Track Milestones after Total Hip Arthroplasty[11]

HSS TOTAL KNEE ARTHROPLASTY-FUNCTIONAL MILESTONES FORM

REHABILITATION DEPARTMENT
PHYSICAL THERAPY
PT Initials: _____
Diagnosis: _____ Age: _____
Right/Left/Bilateral
Porous/Hybrid/Cemented
Initial/Revision
WBAT PWB TTWB NWB
Height _____ (in) Weight _____ (lbs) | **Day of Surgery:** Su M T W Th F Sa

Anesthesia: EPI GEN
PCA: EPI IV
Nerve Block: Psoas/Sciatic/None

Pre-op class: YES NO
Pre-op Amb: w/c bound <1 1–5 6–10 >10 Blocks
Pre-op Assistive Device: Cane/Crutches/Walker/None
Need to negotiate stairs: YES NO
Pre-op Lives Alone: YES NO

BID																
Discharge																
Stairs Unassisted																
Stairs Aassisted																
Cane Unassisted																
Cane Aassisted																
Walker Unassisted																
Walker Aassisted																
Stand Only																
Transfer Unassisted																
Transfer Assisted																
Pain Level																
Date of Surgery _____																
P.O.D.	RR	1	2	3	4	5	6	7	8	9	10	11	12	13	14	15

Discharge To: Home   Rehab   SNF
If D/c to home: Home PT   Outpatient   No PT
If D/c to home, with: Family/Friends/Other   Alone

Complications/PT Held: _____
_____
_____
_____

continued on next page

PERTINENT PAST MEDICAL HISTORY
Please circle all that apply

Cardiovascular
1. A-fib/arrythmia
2. Angina
3. CAD
4. ↑ Cholesterol
5. HTN
6. MI
7. Tachycardia
8. Valve disease

Circulatory
9. Cellulitis
10. DVT
11. PVD
12. Phlebitis
13. PE

Endocrine
14. DM
15. Hyperthyroidism
16. Hypothyroidism
17. Renal disease

Hearing/Vision
18. Blind
19. Glaucoma
20. Cataracts
21. HOH
22. Deaf

Immunological/Infectious Disease
23. Chronic Infection
24. HIV
25. Hepatitis

Musculoskeletal
26. AVN
27. DDD
   Fractures
28. -Femur
29. -Pelvis
30. -Spine
31. -Humerus
32. -Wrist
33. -Other
34. HO
35. HNP
36. LBackP
37. OA
38. OP
39. Rotator cuff tear
40. Sciatica
41. Scoliosis
42. Spinal stenosis

Neurological
43. Alzheimers/dementia
44. CP
45. CVA/TIA
46. MS
47. Parkinsons
48. Paraparesis
49. Paraplegia
50. Polio
51. RSD
52. Seizures

Oncology
Cancer
53. -Breast
54. -Colon
55. -Leukemia
56. -Lung
57. -Lymphoma
58. -Prostate
59. -Other malignant

Psychological
60. Anxiety/panic
29. Bipolar dsorder
30. Depression
31. Schizophrenia

Pulmonary
64. Asthma
65. CHF
66. COPD/emphysema
67. Pneumonia
68. SOB

Rheumatological
69. Fibromyalgia
70. JRA
71. SLE
72. Psoriatic arthritis
73. RA

Other
74. Drug/substance abuse
75. Mental retardation
76. Obesity
77. Ulcer disease/gastric

Other PMH:
78. _____
_____
_____
_____
_____

PAST SURGICAL HISTORY

79. TKR
80. TKR revision
81. THR
82. THR revision
83. TSR

84. Spine
85. Arthroscopy -LE
86. Arthroscopy -UE
87. Amputee UE
88. Amputee LE
89. ORIF UE
90. ORIF LE

91. Ligament/joint reconstrucion
92. CABG
93. Pacemaker
94. Valve replacement
95. Recent major abdominal surgery (within last 6 months)

Other PSH:
96. _____
_____
_____
_____

Phases of Cardiac Rehabilitation

Phase I: Acute Phase or Monitoring Phase	Inpatient cardiac rehabilitation begins when the patient is determined to be medically stable after a myocardial infarction, coronary artery bypass surgery, angioplasty, valve repair, or congestive heart failure.
Phase II: Subacute Phase of Rehabilitation or Conditioning Phase	This initial outpatient phase begins as early as 24 hours after discharge, and lasts up to 6 weeks. Frequency of visits depends on the patient's clinical needs. Patients are monitored by electrocardiogram telemetry and are taught the basics of self-monitoring and proper exercise procedure. In addition, secondary prevention of disease by implementation of risk factor reduction is a key component of this phase.
Phase III: Training or Intensive Rehabilitation	Patients are usually seen once a week, and training or rehabilitation extends from the time the patient finishes phase II to indefinitely. Patients exercise in larger groups and continue to progress in their exercise program. Resistance training often begins in this phase.
Phase IV: Ongoing Conditioning (Maintenance) Phase or Prevention Program	Candidates for this program are individuals who are at high risk for infarction because of their risk-factor profile, as well as those who want to continue to be followed by supervision of trained personnel.

Tools for Practice

Health Care and the Law[7,21,54,55]

Federal statutes address those areas the federal government is constitutionally permitted to regulate, such as interstate commerce and taxation. Federal statutes apply consistently to all citizens across state lines and, where they conflict with related state laws, generally supersede state law. A number of federal statutes may affect the provision of physical therapy services, including the following:

The Americans with Disabilities Act (ADA)	Requires that goods and services (including health care) available to the public are accessible to persons with disabilities. The ADA prohibits discrimination against people with disabilities in employment (Title I), public services (Title II), in places of public accommodation and commercial facilities (Title III), and telecommunications (Title IV). Therapists can assist patients by providing justification for ADA-prescribed reasonable accommodations to employers, insurance companies, and others.
The Individuals with Disabilities Education Act (IDEA)	Requires that special education and related services (including physical therapy) be provided at public expense to students with disabilities when needed for those students to benefit from an education program. The IDEA is a law ensuring services to children with disabilities throughout the nation. IDEA governs how states and public agencies provide early intervention, special education, and related services to more than 6.5 million eligible infants, toddlers, children, and youth with disabilities. Infants and toddlers with disabilities (birth-2 years) and their families receive early intervention services under IDEA Part C. Children and youth (ages 3–21) receive special education and related services under IDEA Part B.
The Social Security Act Amendments of 1965	Contains, among other provisions, the foundation for (1) the Medicare program, a federally subsidized health insurance program for people 65 years and older,[5] and (2) Medicaid, jointly funded by the state and federal governments as a program designed to provide health care services to the poor. Physical therapy is among the health care services reimbursed under Medicare and Medicaid.
The Health Insurance Portability and Accountability Act (HIPAA)	HIPAA includes federal guidelines that protect the confidentiality of health information. Health information is to be shared only with persons authorized to view the information (i.e., professionals involved in providing health care). Facilities assume the responsibility of designing systems to assure that health information is protected and kept confidential. All health care professionals are bound by these guidelines. Therapists must assure that discussions involving patients' health information occur in secure locations.

Vital Signs, Biometrics, and Lab Values

Vital Signs: Normal Ranges [10,39,46,47,49]

Age Group	Respiratory Rate	Heart Rate	Diastolic Blood Pressure	Systolic Blood Pressure	Temperature	Weight (kg)	Weight (lb)
Newborn	30–60	100–160	Varies	20–60	97.7 °F (36.5 °C)	2–3	4.5–7
Infant (1–12 mos)	24–38	90–160	Varies	70–80	98.6 °F (37.0 °C)*	4–10	9–22
Toddler (1–3 yrs)	22–30	80–125	48–80	80–110	98.6 °F (37.0 °C)*	10–14	22–31
Preschooler (3–5 yrs)	20–24	80–115	48–80	80–110	98.6 °F (37.0 °C)*	14–18	31–40
School Age (6–12 yrs)	16–22	60–100	60–64	90–100	98.6 °F (37.0 °C)*	20–42	41–92
Adolescent (13–17 yrs)	14–20	60–100	70–80	100–120	98.6 °F (37.0 °C)*	>50	>110
Adults (18+ yrs)	18–20	60–100	<80	<120	98.6 °F (37.0 °C)*	Varies	Depends on body size

Remember these points:

The patient's normal range should always be taken into consideration.

Heart rate, blood pressure, and respiratory rate are expected to increase during times of fever or stress.

Respiratory rate for infants should be counted for a full 60 seconds.

*Ranges from 97.8 °F to 99.1 °F (36.5 °C to 37.3 °C).

Strength/Weight/Height

Body mass index (BMI) is body weight in kilograms divided by height in meters squared (kg/m^2).

To determine BMI, locate the height of interest in the left-most column and read across the row for that height to the weight of interest. Follow the column of the weight up to the top row that lists the BMI. A BMI of 18.5 to 24.9 is the healthy-weight range, BMI of 25 to 29.9 is the overweight range, and BMI of 30 and above is in the obese range.

BMI	19	20	21	22	23	24	25	26	27	28	29	30	31	32	33	34	35
Height							Weight in Pounds										
4'10"	91	96	100	105	110	115	119	124	129	134	138	143	148	153	158	162	167
4'11"	94	99	104	109	114	119	124	128	133	138	143	148	153	158	163	168	173
5'	97	102	107	112	118	123	128	133	138	143	148	153	158	163	158	174	179
5'1"	100	106	111	116	122	127	132	137	143	148	153	158	164	169	174	180	185
5'2"	104	109	115	120	126	131	136	142	147	153	158	164	169	175	180	186	191
5'3"	107	113	118	124	130	135	141	146	152	158	163	169	175	180	186	191	197
5'4"	110	116	122	128	134	140	145	151	157	163	169	174	180	186	192	197	204
5'5"	114	120	126	132	138	144	150	156	162	168	174	180	186	192	198	204	210
5'6"	118	124	130	136	142	148	155	161	167	173	179	186	192	198	204	210	216
5'7"	121	127	134	140	146	153	159	166	172	178	185	191	198	204	211	217	223
5'8"	125	131	138	144	151	158	164	171	177	184	190	197	203	210	216	223	230
5'9"	128	135	142	149	155	162	169	176	182	189	196	203	209	216	223	230	236
5'10"	132	139	146	153	160	167	174	181	188	195	202	209	216	222	229	236	243
5'11"	136	143	150	157	165	172	179	186	193	200	208	215	222	229	236	243	250
6'	140	147	154	162	169	177	184	191	199	206	213	221	228	235	242	250	258
6'1"	144	151	159	166	174	182	189	197	204	212	219	227	235	242	250	257	265
6'2"	148	155	163	171	179	186	194	202	210	218	225	233	241	249	256	264	272
6'3"	152	160	168	176	184	192	200	208	216	224	232	240	248	256	264	272	279
	Healthy Weight						Overweight					Obese					

From U.S. Department of Health and Human Services, U.S. Department of Agriculture: *Dietary guidelines for Americans 2005*, ed 6, Washington, DC, 2005, Authors. Accessible at *www.healthierus.gov/dietaryguidelines*.

Source: National Institutes of Health, National Heart, Lung, and Blood Institute: *Evidence report of clinical guidelines on the identification, evaluation, and treatment of overweight and obesity in adults*, Bethesda, Md, 1998, Author.

BMI

The BMI can be calculated using pounds and inches with this equation:

$$BMI = \frac{\text{Weight in pounds}}{[(\text{Height in inches}) \times (\text{Height in inches})]} \times 703.$$

For example, a person who weighs 220 pounds and is 6 feet 3 inches tall has a BMI of 27.5, based on the following calculation:

$$\frac{220}{[(75\,\text{inches}) \times (75\,\text{inches})]} \times 703 = 27.5.$$

Blood: Normal Ranges and Causes of Abnormal Results[9,67]

Red Blood Cells (RBCs)		SI Units	Causes of Abnormal Results
Adult female	4.0–5.5 million/μL	$4.0–5.5 \times 10^{12}$/L	Increased: Hemoconcentration, dehydration, COPD, CHF, high altitude, polycythemia vera, smokers, cardiovascular disease, congenital heart disease, chronic lung disease, renal cell carcinoma, other erythropoietin-producing neoplasms, stress, hemoconcentration/dehydration
Pregnant	3.0–5.0 million/μL	$3.0–5.0 \times 10^{12}$/L	
Adult male	4.5–6.2 million/μL	$4.5–6.2 \times 10^{12}$/L	
Infant	3.8–6.1 million/μL	$3.8–6.1 \times 10^{12}$/L	
1–2 yrs	3.6–5.5 million/μL	$3.6–5.5 \times 10^{12}$/L	
6–15 yrs	4.7–4.8 million/μL	$4.7–4.8 \times 10^{12}$/L	
			Decreased: anemia, hemolysis, chronic renal failure, hemorrhage, marrow failure, Hodgkin disease, lymphoma, multiple myeloma, leukemia, systemic lupus erythematosus (SLE), Addison disease, rheumatic fever, subacute bacterial endocarditis, hyperthyroidism, cirrhosis

White Blood Cells (WBCs)		SI Units	Causes of Abnormal Results
Adult females	4500–11,000/μL	$4.5–11.0 \times 10^{9}$/L	Increased: most commonly related to increased numbers of neutrophils, lymphocytes, eosinophils, or monocytes
Pregnant			
Trimester 1	6600–14,000/μL	$6.6–14.1 \times 10^{9}$/L	
Trimester 2	6900–17,100/μL	$6.9–17.1 \times 10^{9}$/L	Decreased: viral infections, hypersplenism, bone marrow suppression due to drugs (e.g., antimetabolites, barbiturates, antibiotics, antihistamines, anticonvulsants, antithyroid meds, arsenicals, cancer chemotherapy, cardiovascular drugs/analgesics, antiinflammatory drugs), primary bone marrow disorders (leukemia, myeloma, aplastic anemia, congenital disorders, myelodysplastic syndromes), immune-associated neutropenia, marrow-occupying diseases (fungal infection, metastatic tumor)
Trimester 3	5900–14,700/μL	$5.9–14.7 \times 10^{9}$/L	
Postpartum	9700–25,700/μL	$9.7–25.7 \times 10^{9}$/L	
Adult males	4500–11,000/μL	$4.5–11.0 \times 10^{9}$/L	
Children			
Newborn	9000–30,000/μL	$9.0–30.0 \times 10^{9}$/L	
3 mos	5700–18,000/μL	$5.7–18.0 \times 10^{9}$/L	
1 yr	6000–17,500/μL	$6.0–17.5 \times 10^{9}$/L	
3 yrs	5700–16,300/μL	$5.7–16.3 \times 10^{9}$/L	
10 yrs	4500–13,500/μL	$4.5–13.5 \times 10^{9}$/L	

White Blood Cells (WBCs)		SI Units	Causes of Abnormal Results
Differential WBCs			
Granulocytes			
Segmented neutrophils (Segs)	40%–75%	0.40–0.75	Increased: acute bacterial infections, tissue breakdown (trauma, burns, tumors, gangrene, acute MI, stress), myelogenous leukemia, hemolysis, uremia, diabetic acidosis, acute gout, seizures, severe exercise, late pregnancy and labor, many drugs
Adults	3800/μL	3800×10^6/L	
Children			
Birth	8400/μL	8400×10^6/L	
12 hrs	12,100/μL	$12,100 \times 10^6$/L	
24 hrs	8870/μL	8870×10^6/L	
1 wk	4100/μL	4100×10^6/L	
2 wks	3320/μL	3320×10^6/L	
1–2 mos	2750/μL	2750×10^6/L	
4 mos	2730/μL	2730×10^6/L	
6 mos	2710/μL	2710×10^6/L	
8 mos	2680/μL	2680×10^6/L	
10 mos	2600/μL	2600×10^6/L	
12 mos	2680/μL	2680×10^6/L	
2 yrs	2660/μL	2660×10^6/L	
4 yrs	3040/μL	3040×10^6/L	
6 yrs	3600/μL	3600×10^6/L	
8–14 yrs	3700/μL	3700×10^6/L	
16–20 yrs	3800/μL	3800×10^6/L	
Band Neutrophils (Bands)			
Proportion	0%–10%	0.00–0.10	Decreased: viral infections, aplastic anemia, agranulocytosis, immunosuppressive drugs, radiation therapy to bone marrow, drugs (e.g., antibiotics, antithyroid drugs), lymphocytic and monocytic leukemias
Adults	620/μL	620×10^6/L	
Children			
Birth	2540/μL	2540×10^6/L	
12 hrs	3460/μL	3460×10^6/L	
24 hrs	2680/μL	2680×10^6/L	
1 wk	1420/μL	1420×10^6/L	
2 wks	1200/μL	1200×10^6/L	
1 mo	1150/μL	1150×10^6/L	
2 mos	1100/μL	1100×10^6/L	
4–10 mos	1000/μL	1000×10^6/L	
12 mos	990/μL	990×10^6/L	
2 yrs	850/μL	850×10^6/L	
4 yrs	710/μL	710×10^6/L	
6 yrs	670/μL	670×10^6/L	
8 yrs	660/μL	660×10^6/L	

Continued

White Blood Cells (WBCs)		SI Units	Causes of Abnormal Results
10 yrs	645/μL	645 × 10⁶/L	
12–14 yrs	640/μL	640 × 10⁶/L	
16–20 yrs	620/μL	620 × 10⁶/L	
Eosinophils (Eos)			
Proportion	0%–5%	0.00–0.05	Increased: allergies, eczema, contact dermatitis, reactions to certain drugs (e.g., iodides, sulfa drugs, chlorpromazine), chronic granulomatous diseases (sarcoidosis), parasitic infections, lymphomas, lung cancer, pulmonary infiltrates with eosinophilia (PIE), hypereosinophilic syndrome, polycythemia, subacute infections, polyarteritis nodosa, inflammatory bowel diseases
Adults	200/μL	200 × 10⁶/L	
Children			
Birth	400/μL	400 × 10⁶/L	
12–24 hrs	450/μL	450 × 10⁶/L	
1 wk	500/μL	500 × 10⁶/L	
2 wks	350/μL	350 × 10⁶/L	
1 mo–1 yr	300/μL	300 × 10⁶/L	
2 yrs	80/μL	280 × 10⁶/L	Decreased: adrenal steroid production due to bodily stress (burns, postsurgery, SLE), acute infections, infectious mononucleosis, congestive heart failure (CHF), Cushing's syndrome, drugs (e.g., adrenocorticotropic hormone, epinephrine, throxine, prostaglandins), infections with neutrophilia, neutropenia
4 yrs	250/μL	250 × 10⁶/L	
6 yrs	230/μL	230 × 10⁶/L	
8–20 yrs	200/μL	200 × 10⁶/L	
Basophils (Basos)			
Proportion	0%–1%	0.0–0.01	Increased: leukemia, inflammatory processes, polycythemia vera, Hodgkin's disease, hemolytic anemia following splenectomy or radiation therapy, myeloid metaplasia
Adults	40/μL	40 × 10⁶/L	
Children			
Birth–24 hrs	100/μL	100 × 10⁶/L	
1 wk–8 yrs	50/μL	50 × 10⁶/L	Decreased: stress reactions (acute myocardial infarction, bleeding ulcer), hypersensitivity reactions, steroids, pregnancy, hyperthyroidism
10–20 yrs	40/μL	40 × 10⁶/L	
Monocytes (Monos)			
Proportion	2%–14%	0.02–0.14	Increased: viral diseases, recovery phase of various acute infections, neoplasms, disseminated tuberculosis, inflammatory bowel disease, subacute bacterial endocarditis, collagen diseases, hematologic disorders (AML, CML, polycythemia vera, lymphoma, multiple myeloma)
Adults	300/μL	300 × 10⁶/L	
Children			
Birth	1050/μL	1050 × 10⁶/L	
12 hrs	1200/μL	1200 × 10⁶/L	
24 hrs–1 wk	1100/μL	1100 × 10⁶/L	
2 wks	1000/μL	1000 × 10⁶/L	
1 mo	700/μL	700 × 10⁶/L	Decreased: aplastic anemia, lymphocytic leukemias, hairy cell leukemia, prednisone, RA, HIV
2 mos	650/μL	650 × 10⁶/L	
4 mos	600/μL	600 × 10⁶/L	
6–8 mos	580/μL	580 × 10⁶/L	

White Blood Cells (WBCs)		SI Units	Causes of Abnormal Results
10–12 mos	550/μL	550×10^6/L	
2 yrs	530/μL	530×10^6/L	
4 yrs	450/μL	450×10^6/L	
6 yrs	400/μL	400×10^6/L	
8–12 yrs	350/μL	350×10^6/L	
14 yrs	380/μL	380×10^6/L	
16–18 yrs	400/μL	400×10^6/L	
20 yrs	380/μL	380×10^6/L	
Lymphocytes (Lymphs)			
Proportion	25%–40%	0.25–0.40	Increased: chronic infections, infectious mononucleosis and other viral infections (cytomegalovirus, upper respiratory infections, etc.), lymphocytic leukemias, ulcerative colitis, hypoadrenalism, immunogenic thrombocytopenic purpura
Adults	2500/μL	2500×10^6/L	
Children			
Birth-12 hrs	5500/μL	5500×10^6/L	
24 hrs	5800/μL	5800×10^6/L	
1 wk	5000/μL	5000×10^6/L	
2 wks	5500/μL	5500×10^6/L	Decreased: AIDS-related complex, bone marrow suppression from chemotherapy, aplastic anemia, neoplasms, steroids, adrenocortical hyperfunction, neurological disorders (multiple sclerosis, myasthenia gravis, Guillain-Barré syndrome), SLE, burns, trauma, chronic uremia, tuberculosis, Cushing syndrome
1 mo	6000/μL	6000×10^6/L	
2 mos	6300/μL	6300×10^6/L	
4 mos	6800/μL	6800×10^6/L	
6 mos	7300/μL	7300×10^6/L	
8 mos	7600/μL	7600×10^6/L	
10 mos	7500/μL	7500×10^6/L	
12 mos	7000/μL	7000×10^6/L	
2 yrs	6300/μL	6300×10^6/L	
4 yrs	4500/μL	4500×10^6/L	
6 yrs	3500/μL	3500×10^6/L	
8 yrs	3300/μL	3300×10^6/L	
10 yrs	3100/μL	3100×10^6/L	
12 yrs	3000/μL	3000×10^6/L	
14 yrs	2900/μL	2900×10^6/L	
16 yrs	2800/μL	2800×10^6/L	
18 yrs	2700/μL	2700×10^6/L	
20 yrs	2500/μL	2500×10^6/L	

Urinalysis Results[9]

Albumin	Negative
Appearance	Clear to faintly hazy
Bilirubin	Negative
Color	Yellow
Glucose or reducing substances	Negative
Ketones	Negative
Leukocyte esterase	Negative
Nitrite	Negative
Occult blood	Negative
Odor	Faint (not fruity, musty, fishy, or fetid)
pH	4.5–8.0
Protein	Negative
Specific gravity	1.003–1.030
Urobilinogen	Negative or 0.1–1 Ehrlich U/dl
Cells	
Erythrocytes	< 3 cells/HPF
Leukocytes	≤4 cells/HPF
Urinary tract epithelium	≤10 cells/HPF
Casts	Moderate clear protein casts
Crystals	Small amount
Bacteria or fungi	None or < 1000/ml
Parasites	None

Coding and Billing

Common CPT Codes

Note: This list of codes may not be all-inclusive.

COVERED WHEN MEDICALLY NECESSARY:

CPT* Codes	Description
97001	Physical therapy evaluation
97002	Physical therapy reevaluation
97010	Application of a modality to one or more areas; hot or cold packs
97012	Application of a modality to one or more areas; traction, mechanical
97014	Application of a modality to one or more areas; electrical stimulation (unattended)

CPT* Codes	Description
97016	Application of a modality to one or more areas; vasopneumatic devices
97018	Application of a modality to one or more areas; paraffin bath
97022	Application of a modality to one or more areas; whirlpool
97024	Application of a modality to one or more areas; diathermy (e.g., microwave)
97026	Application of a modality to one or more areas; infrared
97028	Application of a modality to one or more areas; ultraviolet
97032	Application of a modality to one or more areas; electrical stimulation (manual), each 15 minutes
97033	Application of a modality to one or more areas; iontophoresis, each 15 minutes
97034	Application of a modality to one or more areas; contrast baths, each 15 minutes
97035	Application of a modality to one or more areas; ultrasound, each 15 minutes
97036	Application of a modality to one or more areas; Hubbard tank, each 15 minutes
97110	Therapeutic procedure, one or more areas, each 15 minutes; therapeutic exercises to develop strength and endurance, range of motion, and flexibility
97112	Therapeutic procedure, one or more areas, each 15 minutes; neuromuscular reeducation of movement, balance, coordination, kinesthetic sense, posture, and/or proprioception for sitting and/or standing activities
97113	Therapeutic procedure, one or more areas, each 15 minutes; aquatic therapy with therapeutic exercises
97116	Therapeutic procedure, one or more areas, each 15 minutes; gait training (includes stair climbing)
97124	Therapeutic procedure, one or more areas, each 15 minutes; massage, including effleurage, pétrissage and/or tapotement (stroking, compression, percussion)
97140	Manual therapy techniques (e.g., mobilization/manipulation, manual lymphatic drainage, manual traction), one or more regions, each 15 minutes
97530	Therapeutic activities, direct (one-on-one) patient contact by the provider (use of dynamic activities to improve functional performance), each 15 minutes
97535	Self-care/home management training (e.g., activities of daily living [ADL] and compensatory training, meal preparation, safety procedures, and instructions in use of assistive technology devices/adaptive equipment), direct one-on-one contact by provider, each 15 minutes
97542	Wheelchair management (e.g., assessment, fitting, training), each 15 minutes
97760	Orthotic(s) management and training (including assessment and fitting when not otherwise reported), upper extremity(s), lower extremity(s) and/or trunk, each 15 minutes
97761	Prosthetic training, upper and/or lower extremity(s), each 15 minutes
97762	Checkout for orthotic/prosthetic use, established patient, each 15 minutes

*Current Procedural Terminology (CPT) ©2007 American Medical Association: Chicago, IL.

Common PT- and OT-Related ICD-9 Codes

Ambulation—Gait, Coordination, Balance, and Posture-Related Diagnoses

Diagnosis	ICD-9 Codes
Abnormality of gait: ataxic, paralytic, spastic, staggering	781.2
Cerebral ataxia	331.89
Coordination disorder (clumsiness, dyspraxia, and/or specific motor development disorder)	315.4
Difficulty in walking	719.70
Friedreich ataxia	334.0
Lack of coordination; ataxia, not otherwise specified; muscular incoordination	781.3
Other cerebellar ataxia	334.3
Other extrapyramidal disease and abnormal movement disorder	333.9

Spine and Related Diagnoses

Adolescent postural kyphosis	737.0
Anomalies of spine	756.10
Back disorders, other unspecified ankylosis of spine, not otherwise specified; compression of spinal nerve root, not elsewhere classified; spinal disorder, not otherwise specified	724.9
Curvature of spine unspecified	737.40
Kyphoscoliosis and scoliosis	737.30
Kyphosis (acquired)	737.10
Lordosis (acquired)	737.20
Lumbago: low back pain, low back syndrome, lumbalgia	724.2
Spina bifida	741.90
Sprains and strains of lumbosacral region	846.0
Sprains and strains of neck	847.0
Sprains and strains of other and unspecified parts of back	847.9
Sprains and strains of sacroiliac region	846.9

Upper Extremity and Related Diagnoses

Diagnosis	ICD-9 Codes
Carpal tunnel syndrome	354.0
Claw hand (acquired)	736.06
Club hand (acquired)	736.07
Clubbing of the fingers	781.5
Contracture of palmer fascia; Dupuytren contracture	728.6
Dislocation of shoulder	831.00
Dislocation of wrist	833.00
Fracture of carpal bones	814.00
Fracture of humerus	812.20
Fracture of radius and ulna	813.83
Injury to brachial plexus (birth trauma—newborn)	767.6
Lower end of forearm: Colles fracture closed	813.41
Swelling of limb	729.81
Wrist drop	736.05

Lower Extremity and Related Diagnoses	
Contracture of joint, lower leg	718.46
Contracture of joint, pelvic region and thigh	718.45
Contracture of tendon (sheath) short Achilles tendon (acquired)	727.81
Swelling of limb	729.81

Bone (Fractures, Dislocations, etc.), Muscle, Joint, Tendon, Fascia, Synovium, Nerve, and Bursa-Related Diagnosis	
Ankylosis of joint	718.50
Contracture of joint, site unspecified	718.40
Disorders of muscle, ligament, and fascia	728.89
Malunion and nonunion of fractures	733.82

Bone (Fractures, Dislocations, etc.), Muscle, Joint, Tendon, Fascia, Synovium, Nerve, and Bursa-Related Diagnosis	
Muscular dystrophy	359.1
Muscular wasting and disuse atrophy	728.2
Other derangement of joint	718.90
Other disorders of bone and cartilage	733.90
Other disorders of muscle, ligament, and fascia	728.89
Other disorders of soft tissue	729.9
Other disorders of synovium, tendon, and bursa	727.89
Other joint derangement, not elsewhere classified *Instability of joint*	718.80
Other musculoskeletal symptoms referable to limbs	729.89
Other specified disorders of joint *Calcification of joint*	719.80
Recurrent dislocation of joints	718.30
Rupture of tendon, nontraumatic	727.60
Spasm of muscle	728.85
Stiffness of joint (unspecified)	719.50
Tendinitis	726.90

Miscellaneous Diagnoses	
Abnormal involuntary movements	781.0
Adult physical abuse	995.81
Alexia and dyslexia	784.61
Birth trauma unspecified	767.9
Blindness	369.00
Chickenpox	052
Chromosomal anomalies: includes syndromes associated with anomalies in the number and form of chromosomes	758.9
Cystic fibrosis	277.00
Deafness	389.9
Edema	782.3
Gout, unspecified	274.9
Head injury, unspecified	959.01
Other acquired deformity	738.9
Rett syndrome	330.8
TBI	854.00
Visual impairment (moderate or severe, both eyes)	369.20
Arithmetic disorder	315.1
Other specific learning difficulties	315.2

American Sign Language[45]

Manual Alphabet

The American Sign Language (ASL) alphabet can be used to communicate effectively with deaf athletes. ASL has short cuts and abbreviations for words or phrases that facilitate communication, but this alphabet shows the basis for the language.

Patient's Checklist Before Exercise Testing or Training Session[21]

- ☐ Feeling well over the past 48 hours
- ☐ No infections (e.g., upper respiratory tract infection) or influenza
- ☐ No temperature
- ☐ No unaccustomed muscle or joint discomfort or pain
- ☐ No chest tightness or pain
- ☐ No unaccustomed breathing difficulty or fatigue
- ☐ Adequate night's sleep
- ☐ Has not eaten heavily within past 3 hours
- ☐ Best time of day
- ☐ Wearing or using orthoses, walking aids, and devices
- ☐ Clothing appropriate for exercise conditions (indoors or outdoors)
- ☐ Appropriate socks, and footwear that is comfortable, well-fitting, and has secured laces (double-knotted)
- ☐ Has water within reach
- ☐ Has taken preexercise medications at specified time
- ☐ Has nitroglycerine within reach (patients with cardiac dysfunction)
- ☐ Has inhaler within reach (patients with pulmonary dysfunction)
- ☐ Has sugar supply within reach (patients with diabetes)
- ☐ Standardize and record the use of orthotics and walking aids

Physical Activity Guidelines for Americans

Age Group	Recommendation	Examples
Children and adolescents	One hour or more of moderate or vigorous aerobic physical activity per day, including vigorous-intensity physical activity at least 3 days a week. Children and adolescents should incorporate muscle-strengthening activities 3 days per week. Bone-strengthening activities are also recommended 3 days per week.	• *Moderate-intensity aerobic activities:* hiking, skateboarding, bicycle riding, and brisk walking • *Vigorous-intensity aerobic activities:* bicycle riding, jumping rope, running, and sports such as soccer, basketball, and ice or field hockey • *Muscle-strengthening activities:* rope climbing, sit-ups, and tug-of-war • *Bone-strengthening activities:* jumping rope, running, and skipping
Adults	Two and one half hours per week of moderate-intensity aerobic physical activity, or 1 hour and 15 minutes of vigorous physical activity. Aerobic activity should be performed in episodes of at least 10 minutes. For more extensive health benefits, adults should increase their aerobic physical activity to 5 hours per week at moderate intensity, or 2.5 hours per week of vigorous-intensity aerobic physical activity. Muscle-strengthening activities at least 2 days per week.	• *Moderate-intensity aerobic activities:* walking briskly, water aerobics, ballroom dancing, and general gardening • *Vigorous-intensity aerobic activities:* racewalking, jogging or running, swimming laps, jumping rope, and hiking uphill or with a heavy backpack • *Muscle-strengthening activities:* weight training, push-ups, sit-ups, and carrying heavy loads or heavy gardening
Older adults	Follow the guidelines for other adults when it is within their physical capacity. If a chronic condition prohibits their ability to follow those guidelines, they should be as physically active as their abilities and conditions allow. If they are at risk of falling, they should also do exercises that maintain or improve balance.	
Women during pregnancy	At least 2.5 hours of moderate-intensity aerobic activity per week during pregnancy and the time after delivery, preferably spread throughout the week. Pregnant women who habitually engage in vigorous aerobic activity or who are highly active can continue during pregnancy and the time after delivery, provided they remain healthy and discuss with their health care provider how and when activity should be adjusted over time.	

Age Group	Recommendation	Examples
Adults with disabilities	At least 2.5 hours of moderate aerobic activity a week, or 1 hour and 15 minutes of vigorous aerobic activity per week. Muscle-strengthening activities involving all major muscle groups 2 or more days per week.	When they are not able to meet the guidelines, they should engage in regular physical activity according to their abilities and should avoid inactivity.
People with chronic medical conditions	Adults with chronic conditions get important health benefits from regular physical activity. They should do so with the guidance of a health care provider.	

For more information about the "Physical Activity Guidelines for Americans," visit www.hhs.gov, or www.health.gov/paguidelines.

Spanish Terminology

Body Parts

Head	Cabeza
Hair	Cabello
Face	Cara
Eyes	Ojos
Nose	Nariz
Ears	Orejas
Lips	Labios
Mouth	Boca
Teeth	Dientes
Tongue	Lengua
Forehead	Frente
Chin	Barbilla
Cheek	Mejilla
Jaw	Mandíbula
Neck	Cuello
Throat	Garganta
Upper back	Parte alta de la espalda
Mid-back	Parte media de la espalda
Low back	Parte baja de la espalda
Shoulder	Hombro
Arm	Brazo
Wrist	Muñeca

Hand	Mano
Finger	Dedo
Thumb	Dedo pulgar
Hip	Cadera
Leg	Pierna
Knee	Rodilla
Ankle	Tobillo
Foot	Pie
Toes	Dedo del pie
Chest	Pecho
Breast	Seno
Stomach	Estómago
Waist	Cintura
Groin	Ingle
Vagina	Vagina
Penis	Pene

Anatomical Terms

Skin	Piel
Bones	Huesos
Muscles	Músculos
Joints	Articulaciones
Skull	Cráneo
Spine	Columna vertebral
Cervical spine	Espina cervical
Thoracic spine	Espina torácica
Lumbar spine	Espina lumbar
Spinal cord	Médula espinal
Vertebrae	Vértebras
Nerves	Nervios
Intervertebral disk	Disco intervertebral
Pelvis	Pelvis
Sacrum	Sacro
Coccyx	Coxis
Vein	Vena
Artery	Arteria
Facet joints	Faceta de las articulaciones
Spinal nerves	Nervios espinales
Anterior/posterior	Anterior/posterior

Patient Prompts

Lie face down	Acuéstese boca abajo
Lie face up	Acuéstese boca arriba
Sit	Siéntese
Stand	Párese
Lie on your side facing me	Acuéstese de lado mirando hacia mí
Other side	Del otro lado
Up	Arriba
Down	Abajo
Relax your head/arm/leg	Relaje su cabeza/brazo/pierna
Inhale deeply	Inhale profundamente
Exhale	Exhale
We are finished	Terminamos
Simple questions	
Do you have pain now?	¿Usted tiene dolor ahora?
Do you have pain here?	¿Usted tiene dolor aquí?
Are you okay?	¿Está bien?
Are you comfortable?	¿Está cómodo?

Symptom Descriptions

Sharp	Agudo
Dull	Sordo
Numb	Adormecido
Shooting	Punzante
Burning	Ardiente
Tingling	Hormigueo
Stabbing	Lancinante
Sore	Irritado
Tight	Tenso
Aching	Doloroso
Weakness	Debilidad
Throbbing	Palpitante

Activities

Standing	Pararse
Sitting	Sentarse

Lying down	Acostarse
Exercise	Ejercitarse
Rest	Descansar
Working	Trabajar
Movement	Movimiento
Lifting	Levantamiento
Bending	Doblarse
Twisting	Torcerse

General Communication

Hello, good morning/afternoon/evening.	Hola, buenos días/buenas tardes/buenas noches.
Welcome to our office.	Bienvenido(a) a nuestra oficina.
Is this your first visit to our clinic?	¿Es ésta su primera visita a nuestra clínica?
Do you have an appointment?	¿Usted tiene una cita?
What is your name?	¿Cuál es su nombre?
Please have a seat, and we will be right with you.	Por favor, tome asiento y estaremos con usted en un momento.
Sorry, I do not speak Spanish.	Discúlpeme, yo no hablo español.
Do you speak English?	¿Usted habla inglés?
One moment please; I will get someone who speaks Spanish.	Un momento por favor. Buscaré a alguien que hable español.
Do you prefer to speak Spanish or English?	¿Usted prefiere hablar en español o en inglés?
Please repeat what you told me.	Repita lo que me dijo, por favor.
I didn't understand you completely. You told me that _____, correct?	No le entendí completamente. ¿Me dijo que _____, correcto?
I still don't understand you.	Todavía no le entiendo.
I didn't understand anything you said to me.	No entendí nada de lo que me dijo.

My Spanish is limited, so please use (simple/everyday) words.	Mi español es limitado, entonces hábleme con palabras (sencillas/comunes).
Please speak more slowly.	Hable más despacio, por favor.
I'm not familiar with that word.	No conozco esa palabra.
What is the meaning of that word?	¿Qué (significa/quiere decir) esa palabra?
I cannot hear you. Please speak louder.	No puedo oírle. Hable más fuerte, por favor.
I did not say that (to you).	No (le) dije eso.
I need a (translator/interpreter)—wait a minute.	Necesito a un (traductor/intérprete)—espere un minuto.
Is this correct?	¿Es esto correcto?
Thank you very much.	Muchas gracias.
You're welcome. (It was nothing.)	De nada. (No fue nada.)
Don't mention it. (You're welcome.)	No hay de que. (De nada.)
It was a pleasure serving you.	Fue un placer haberle atendido.
You are very kind.	Usted es muy amable.
Very nice meeting you.	Mucho gusto en conocerlo(a).
Same to you.	Igualmente.
See you later.	Hasta luego.
Until next time. (See you soon.)	Hasta la próxima vez. (Hasta pronto.)
Goodbye.	Adiós.

Common Conditions

Whiplash	Latigazo
Is a condition caused by a fast stop such as hitting a car or being hit from the rear.	Es una condición causada por una parada súbita tal como al chocar con un auto o al ser chocado por atrás.
Is an injury to the cervical spine or neck.	Es una lesión en la espina cervical o el cuello.

Involves stretched and torn tendons and ligaments.

Symptoms include:
   sore neck
   headache
   difficulty sleeping
   aching in the neck and shoulders

   numbness and tingling in the hands and fingers
   sharp pain in the shoulders and arms
   vision problems
   problems with concentration

Evaluation/examination includes:

   neurological and orthopedic testing
   palpation
   x-ray examination of the area

Rehabilitation includes exercises designed specifically to increase flexibility and strength in the neck.

Involucra estiramiento y desgarre de los tendones y ligamentos.

Los síntomas incluyen:
   dolor de cuello
   dolor de cabeza
   dificultad para dormir
   dolor en el cuello y los hombros
   adormecimiento y hormigueo en las manos y los dedos
   dolor agudo en los hombros y brazos
   problemas en la vista
   problemas de concentración

La evaluación/examinación incluye:
   examinación neurológica y ortopédica
   palpar
   examinación radiográfica del área

La rehabilitación incluye ejercicios diseñados específicamente para aumentar la flexibilidad y la fuerza en el cuello.

Low Back Pain

Is a condition of pain in the low part of the spine near the waist.

The pain:
   may be from a disk (cartilage pad between vertebrae) injury in the lumbar spine (low back).

   may be from strained muscles, ligaments, or tendons in the area.

Dolor En La Parte Baja De La Espalda

Es una condición de dolor en la parte baja de la columna cerca de la cintura.

El dolor:
   puede ser debido a una lesión en un disco (almohadilla de cartílago entre las vértebras) en la columna lumbar (parte baja de la espalda).
   puede ser debido a músculos, ligamentos o tendones estirados en el área.

may run down part of a leg (usually the back of the leg) to the feet and toes.

may cause the person to lean to one side during the early symptoms (do you lean away from the pain or toward the pain?).

Evaluation/examination includes:

palpation
neurological and orthopedic testing

Treatment includes:
muscle massage (deep or superficial)
rehabilitation
education in correct lifting

modification of negative personal habits (e.g., use of tobacco, alcohol, and drugs)

Rehabilitation involves exercises to increase strength and motion.

Sacroiliac/Pelvic Pain

Located in the SI area, small joints between the pelvis and the sacrum, the base of the spine.

Resulting from a misalignment of the joints and stress on the muscles.

Symptoms include pain over the area of the misalignment but not running down the leg.

---

puede extenderse a una parte de una pierna (generalmente la parte de atrás de la pierna) a los pies y dedos de los pies.

puede causar que la persona se incline hacia un lado durante la fase temprana de los síntomas.

¿Usted se inclina hacia el dolor o hacia el lado contrario?

La evaluación/examinación incluye:
palpar
examinación neurológica y ortopédica

El tratamiento incluye:
masajes musculares (profundo o superficial)
rehabilitación
educación acerca del levantamiento correcto
modificación de los hábitos personales negativos (por ejemplo, uso de tabaco, alcohol y drogas)

La rehabilitación incluye ejercicios para aumentar la fuerza y el movimiento.

Dolor Sacroilíaco/Pélvico

Está localizado en el área sacroilíaca, pequeñas articulaciones entre la pelvis y el sacro, la base de la espina.

Resulta de una desalineación de las articulaciones y estrés en los músculos.

Los síntomas incluyen dolor sobre el área de la desalineación pero no se extiende a la pierna.

Evaluation/examination of the problem includes:
palpation (feeling with the hand) of the area of the pain movement or motion of the SI joints

Rehabilitation involves increasing strength and motion.

Cervical/Neck Pain

May have several causes including acute trauma. It may be chronic or have a gradual onset over a long period.

Symptoms include:
sharp or dull pain in the back of the neck or on the right or left side
numbness and tingling in the arm, hand, or fingers
burning sensation in the arm

loss of muscle strength in the arm and hand
pain, possibly located in and caused by muscles in the neck and shoulders

Evaluation/examination of the problem includes:
palpation of the joints and muscles of the painful area of the neck
neurological and orthopedic testing
testing movement/motion in the neck

Rehabilitation of the area to increase strength and motion may involve:
exercise
posture correction
lifestyle changes

La evaluación/examinación del problema incluye:
palpar (sentir con la mano) el área del dolor movimiento de las articulaciones sacroilíacas

La rehabilitación incluye ejercicios para aumentar la fuerza y el movimiento.

Dolor Cervical/De Cuello

Pueden haber varias causas incluyendo trauma agudo, el cual puede ser crónico o comenzar lentamente a través de un largo periodo de tiempo.

Los síntomas incluyen:
dolor agudo o sordo en la parte de atrás del cuello o en el lado izquierdo o derecho
adormecimiento y hormigueo en el brazo, la mano o los dedos
sensación ardiente (de ardor) en el brazo
pérdida de fuerza muscular en el brazo y la mano
dolor, posiblemente localizado y causado por los músculos del cuello y los hombros

La evaluación/examinación del problema incluye:
palpar las articulaciones y los músculos en el área adolorida del cuello
evaluación neurológica y ortopédica
evaluación del movimiento del cuello

La rehabilitación del área para aumentar fortaleza y movimiento puede incluir:
ejercicio
corrección de postura
cambios en el estilo de vida

Muscle Spasm and Pain

Have several causes including acute trauma. Muscle spasm and pain may also be chronic or have a gradual onset over a long period.

Symptoms include (Do you have . . . ?):
sharp or dull pain in the neck

sharp or dull pain in the shoulder
sharp or dull pain in the arm

sharp or dull pain in the back

sharp or dull pain in the buttocks
sharp or dull pain in the leg

Pain may be (Is your pain . . . ?):

spread out
located in a specific area

dull
aching

Evaluation/examination includes palpation of the area and testing of the adjacent body joints.

Treatment includes:
cold when pain is acute

heat when pain is chronic

both heat and cold in long-standing cases
deep massage of muscles

Espasmos Y Dolores Musculares

Tienen varias causas incluyendo trauma agudo. Los espasmos y dolores musculares pueden ser crónicos o comenzar lentamente a través de un largo periodo de tiempo.

Los síntomas incluyen (¿Usted tiene . . . ?):
dolor agudo o sordo en el cuello

dolor agudo o sordo en el hombro
dolor agudo o sordo en el brazo

dolor agudo o sordo en la espalda

dolor agudo o sordo en las nalgas
dolor agudo o sordo en la pierna

El dolor puede ser (¿Su dolor es . . . ?):
esparcido
localizado en un área específica

sordo
doloroso

La evaluación/examinación incluye palpar el área y examinar las articulaciones circundantes.

El tratamiento incluye:
frío cuando el dolores es agudo

calor cuando el dolor es crónico

calor y frío en los casos prolongados
masajes profundos de los músculos

Headache

Causes are:
vascular, neurological, and physiological

Symptoms include pain located in (Where is the pain? Is the pain in/on/or . . . ?):
the front of the head
the back of the head
the sides of the head
deep inside the head
behind the eyes

Pain characteristics include (Is the/there pain . . . ?):
dull
sharp
aching pain
throbbing pain with possible nausea and vomiting
pain with blurred vision
pain with dizziness

Evaluation/examination includes a detailed health history including the following questions about the characteristics of the individual's headache:

Where is the headache, and is it on one side of the head only?

How long have you had the headache?
Do you wake with the pain?
Do you have pain at the end of the day?
Do you have many headaches connected to each other—a cluster?
Is the pain focused on some part of the head?

Neurological testing may be required to find the cause.

Dolor De Cabeza

Las causas son:
vasculares, neurológicas y fisiológicas

Los síntomas incluyen dolor en (¿Dónde está el dolor? ¿El dolor está en/o . . . ?):
el frente de la cabeza
la parte de atrás de la cabeza
los lados de la cabeza
profundo en la cabeza
detrás de los ojos

Las características del dolor incluyen (¿El dolor es . . . ?):
sordo
agudo
doloroso
dolor palpitante posiblemente con náuseas y vómitos
dolor con visión borrosa
dolor con mareos

La evaluación/examinación incluye un historial detallado incluyendo las siguientes preguntas acerca de las características del dolor de cabeza de la persona:

¿Dónde está el dolor de cabeza y si está es un solo lado de la cabeza?

¿Cuánto tiempo lleva con el dolor de cabeza?
¿Se despierta con el dolor?
¿Tiene el dolor al final del día?

¿Padece de muchos dolores de cabeza conectados unos a otro?

¿El dolor está enfocado en una parte de la cabeza?

Puede requerirse examinación neurológica para encontrar la causa.

Ruling out certain diagnoses is also important because there may be a more serious cause for the headache.

También es importante descartar ciertos diagnósticos porque pueden haber causas más serias que producen el dolor de cabeza.

Treatment may include:
deep massage of neck and shoulder muscles

use of heat or cold packs on adjacent areas

exercise associated with the treatment

Therapy may include the use of electrical/nonelectrical devices.

El tratamiento puede incluir:
masajes profundos de los músculos del cuello y los hombros
uso de compresas frías o calientes en las áreas adyacentes
ejercicio asociado con el tratamiento

La terapia puede incluir el uso de aparatos eléctricos/no eléctricos.

Degenerative Joint Pain

Dolor En La Articulación Degenerativo

Caused by deterioration of the joint structure, sometimes with an accumulation of calcium or extra bone in or near the joint.

Es causado por el deterioro de la estructura de la articulación, algunas veces con la acumulación de calcio o hueso adicional en o alrededor de la articulación.

Causes include acute injuries to extremity with a joint and/or soft-tissue effect.

Las causas incluyen lesiones agudas a las extremidades con un efecto en la articulación y/o tejido blando.

Located in the extremities of the body including (Do you have pain in the . . . ?):
shoulder
elbow
wrist/hand/fingers

hip
knee
ankle
feet/toes

Está localizado en las extremidades del cuerpo incluyendo (¿Usted tiene dolor en . . . ?):
el hombro
el codo
la muñeca/la mano/los dedos de las manos
la cadera
la rodilla
el tobillo
los pies/los dedos de los pies

Symptoms include pain in the affected area.	Los síntomas incluyen dolor en el área afectada.
Symptoms in the area of the strain/sprain include:	Los síntomas en el área de torcedura/dislocadura incluyen:
tenderness and soreness over the area	sensibilidad y dolor sobre el área
possible swelling over the area	inflamación posible sobre el área
Pain characteristics include:	Las características de dolor incluyen:
deep aching pain	dolor profundo
burning pain	dolor ardiente
throbbing pain	dolor punzante
sharp pain	dolor agudo
Have you had episodes of arthritis-type joint pain before?	¿Usted ha tenido episodios de algún dolor parecido a la artritis anteriormente?
Areas affected by this pain include (Have you had pain in the . . . ?):	Las áreas afectadas por este dolor incluyen (¿Usted ha tenido este dolor en . . . ?):
neck	el cuello
spine	la espina
joints of the arms, wrists, and fingers	las articulaciones de los brazos, las muñecas y los dedos
joints of the hips, knees, feet, and toes	las articulaciones de las caderas, las rodillas, los pies y los dedos de los pies
Sports participation (In what sports have you ever participated? And for how long?):	Participación deportiva (¿Qué deportes ha prácticado? ¿Y por cuánto tiempo?):
Have you played soccer?	¿Usted ha practicado fútbol?
Have you played football (American with contact)?	¿Usted ha practicado fútbol americano con contacto?
Have you played tennis?	¿Usted ha jugado tenis?
Have you played basketball?	¿Usted ha jugado baloncesto?
Have you played golf?	¿Usted ha jugado golf?
Have you been a runner?	¿Usted ha sido un corredor?
Other?	¿Otro?

Present sports participation (In what sports do you participate now? Any of those I just mentioned?)	Participación deportiva actual (¿Qué deportes practica ahora? ¿Algunos de los que ya mencioné?)
Evaluation/examination includes:	La evaluación/examinación incluye:
palpation of the painful area	palpar el área adolorida
palpation (feeling with the hand) of the area of the pain	palpar (sentir con la mano) el área del dolor
movement of the SI joints	movimiento de las articulaciones sacroilíacas
x-ray examination of the area	examinación radiográfica del área
testing of movement of the painful area	examinación del movimiento del área adolorida
x-ray examination of the painful area	examinación radiográfica del área adolorida
orthopedic and neurological testing of the painful area	evaluación ortopédica y neurológica del área adolorida
Treatment includes:	El tratamiento incluye:
mobilization of the affected joints	movilización de las articulaciones afectadas
massage of the surrounding muscles and other soft tissues	masaje de los músculos y otros tejidos blandos adyacentes
moderate exercise within pain tolerance to increase flexibility and strength	ejercicio moderado dentro de las tolerancias del dolor para aumentar la fortaleza y flexibilidad
Rehabilitation includes increasing strength/motion.	La rehabilitación incluye aumentar la fortaleza/el movimiento.

Carpal Tunnel Syndrome	**Síndrome Del Túnel Carpal**
Defined as a complex of symptoms in the hand and fingers caused by pressure on the median nerve at the wrist.	Se define como un complejo de síntomas en las manos y los dedos de las manos causado por presión sobre el nervio central en la muñeca.

Generally, the cause is some repetitive activity or age degeneration. However, the cause may be unknown.

Symptoms of the condition include:

numbness and tingling of fingers 3, 4, and 5 (Do you have numbness/tingling of fingers 3, 4, and 5?)

nighttime waking with numb hand/fingers (Do you have nighttime waking with numbness in your hand/fingers?)

loss of hand grip strength (Do you have loss of grip strength?)

loss of feeling in the fingers (Do you have loss of feeling in your fingers?)

muscle wasting in hand (Do you have muscle wasting in your hand in the thenar muscle near the thumb?)

Examination/evaluation includes: health history of activities of work and leisure over time

What kind of physical activity have you done for the last 10 years?
What hobbies have you had?
Have you given birth in the last 10 years (if female)?

Generalmente, la causa es algún tipo de actividad repetitiva o degeneración por edad. Sin embargo, la causa puede ser desconocida.

Los síntomas de la condición incluyen:

adormecimiento y hormigueo en los dedos 3, 4 y 5 (¿Usted tiene adormecimiento/hormigueo de los dedos 3, 4 y 5?)

despertarse en medio de la noche con la mano/los dedos de las manos adormecidos. (¿Usted se despierta en medio de la noche con la mano/los dedos de las manos adormecidos?)

pérdida de fuerza de agarre en las manos (¿Usted ha perdido su fuerza de agarre?)

pérdida de sensación en los dedos de las manos (¿Usted ha perdido sensación en los dedos de las manos?)

desgaste del músculo en la mano (¿Usted tiene desgaste muscular en su mano en el músculo de la palma de la mano cerca del dedo pulgar?)

La evaluación/examinación incluye: historial de salud de actividades de trabajo y placer a través del tiempo
¿Qué tipo de actividad física de trabajo ha hecho en los últimos 10 años?
¿Qué pasatiempos ha tenido?
¿Usted ha tenido hijos en los últimos 10 años (si es mujer)?

Examination of orthopedic and neurological signs includes:

sensitivity of hand and fingers (Do you have normal sensitivity of hand and fingers to touch?)

grip strength of hand (Do you have normal strength of hand in response to testing?)

pinch strength of fingers (Do you have normal pinch grip strength in fingers?)

point sensitivity of fingers (Do you have normal point sensitivity in your fingers?)

Treatment includes:
massage of the surrounding muscles and other soft tissues, especially in the forearm and the affected hand
exercise of the wrist and muscles in the forearm to counter stress from overactivity

rest from stressful activity for the affected wrist and arm to allow for healing

Rehabilitation includes flexibility and strengthening exercises, especially exercises opposing normal activities (i.e., exercise in the opposite direction from normal use).

La examinación de los signos ortopédicos y neurológicos incluyen:
sensibilidad en las manos y los dedos de las manos (¿Usted tiene sensibilidad al tacto normal en las manos y los dedos de las manos?)
fuerza de agarre en la mano (¿Usted tiene una fuerza normal en la mano en respuesta a la evaluación?)
fuerza de pinchar en los dedos de las manos (¿Usted tiene una fuerza de agarre de pinza normal en los dedos de las manos?)
sensibilidad en la punta de los dedos (¿Usted tiene una sensibilidad en la punta de los dedos de las manos?)

El tratamiento incluye:
masaje de los músculos y otros tejidos blandos circundantes, especialmente en el antebrazo y mano afectada
ejercicio de la muñeca y los músculos del antebrazo para contrarrestar el estrés de la sobreactividad
descanso de actividades estresantes para la muñeca y el brazo afectado para permitir curación

La rehabilitación incluye ejercicios de flexibilidad y fortalecimiento, especialmente ejercicios opuestos a la actividad normal (por ejemplo, ejercicios en dirección opuesta al uso normal).

Sacroiliac Joint Problems

Causes include misalignment of the pelvis or SI joints. Problems may also originate from disease in or damage to an internal organ.

Located in the SI area, small joints between the pelvis and the sacrum, the base of the spine.

Resulting from a misalignment of the joints and stress on the muscles.

Symptoms include pain over the area of the misalignment but not running down the leg.
Evaluation/examination of the problem includes:
palpation (feeling with the hand) of the area of the pain
movement of the SI joints
x-ray examination of the area

Problemas De Articulación Sacroilíacos

Las causas incluyen desalineación de las articulaciones pélvicas o sacroilíacas. Los problemas también pueden originarse en enfermedad o daño a un órgano interno.

Está localizado en el área sacroilíaca, pequeñas articulaciones entre la pelvis y el sacro, la base de la espina.

Resulta de una desalineación de las articulaciones y tensión en los músculos.

Los síntomas incluyen dolor sobre el área de la desalineación pero no se extiende a la pierna.
La evaluación/examinación del problema incluye:
palpar (sentir con la mano) el área del dolor movimiento de las articulaciones sacroilíacas examinación radiográfica del área

Nonmusculoskeletal Problems

Defined as organic problems in the body and concerned with an organ system.

The cause could be any kind of disease or damage, ranging from an upset stomach to cancer of the liver or some other organ.

Symptoms of the condition range from mild pain to complete dysfunction.

Problemas No Musculoesqueléticos

Se define como problemas orgánicos en el cuerpo y atañe con un sistema de órgano.

La causa puede ser cualquier tipo de enfermedad o daño, que varía desde problemas estomacales hasta cáncer del hígado o algún otro órgano.

Los síntomas de la condición varían desde dolor leve hasta disfunción total.

Examination/evaluation includes consideration of all organs in the body that may be related to the problem and may include laboratory and other tests to determine the cause and the extent of the condition.	La evaluación/examinación incluye consideración de todos los órganos del cuerpo que puedan estar relacionados al problema y puede incluir análisis de laboratorio y otras pruebas para determinar la causa y la extensión de la condición.
Recovery from the problem requires rest and time to heal.	La recuperación para el problema requiere descanso y tiempo para curarse.
Referral is recommended if the treatment is not sufficiently effective in correcting the primary problem within a reasonable amount of time.	Se recomienda referir si el tratamiento no es suficientemente efectivo en corregir el problema principal dentro de un tiempo razonable.
Other treatment may include medications and sometimes surgery.	Otro tratamiento puede incluir medicamentos y en algunas ocasiones cirugía.

Drug Monographs

Introduction to Pharmacology
ACE Inhibitors
α Agonists
α Antagonists or Blockers
Alternative Medications
Angiotensin II Receptor Antagonists
Antiarrhythmics
Antiasthmatics
Antibacterials
Anticholinergics
Anticonvulsants
Antidepressants
Antiemetics
Antifungals
Antihelminthics

Antihistaminics
Antilipidemics
Antineoplastics
Antiprotozoals
Antipsychotics
Antivirals
Anxiolytics
β Agonists
β Antagonists or Blockers
Calcium Channel Blockers
Cholinergic Agonists
CNS Dopaminergic Agonists
Corticosteroids
Diuretics
Drugs and Blood Clotting

Introduction to Pharmacology

Drug

A drug is a chemical that the Food and Drug Administration (FDA) allows the *medical profession* to use to diagnose, prevent, or treat *diseases*. This permission is granted only after the drug company has demonstrated that the drug is *effective and relatively safe* through both animal studies and human clinical trials.

Alternative medications such as herbal preparations are treated as food, and the manufacturer is required to state only content, not amounts, and does not have to provide scientific or clinical proof of efficacy or toxicity. Unsubstantiated claims, varying amounts, and fraud are often encountered with alternative medications.

Drug Name

A drug has three names, but only the last two are used medically:

- Chemical name (e.g., 7-chloro-1,3-dihydro-1-methyl-5-phenyl-2H-1,4-benzodiazepin-2-one)
- Generic or scientific name (e.g., diazepam—only one generic name per drug; often written in parentheses after brand name)

- Brand name (e.g., Valium—there can be different brand names for the same generic drug)

Brand Name *versus* Generic Drug

A brand name drug is the original drug manufactured by a company under a specific brand name, both as a patent is in force and also after the patent has expired.

A generic drug is manufactured by other companies after the patent has expired. A generic drug is a copy that is the same as a brand name drug in composition, dosage, safety, strength, how it is taken, performance, and intended use. It contains the same active ingredient and must show same bioavailability; however, it may have a different appearance. They are usually interchangeable, although a physician may recommend using the brand name drug only.

Therapeutic Considerations of Drug Action

Therapeutic effects are the intended beneficial actions.

Adverse effects are unwanted actions and:

- Must be evaluated as to possibility and more importantly probability
- Can range from mild to severe
- Can be reversible or irreversible
- Can be avoidable (caused by mistake) or unavoidable
- Can often be reduced or reversed when recognized early

Adverse reactions can be classified as:

- Side effects that are associated with a specific drug, are seen in all individuals at different degrees, and are often predictable
- Idiosyncratic reactions that are caused by a biochemical peculiarity of an individual, which becomes apparent only after drug exposure, are seen only in a few patients, do not involve the immune system, and are unpredictable
- Allergic reactions that are caused by an immunological peculiarity of the individual, which becomes apparent only after drug exposure; are seen only in a few patients; and are not necessarily predictable

Placebo

A placebo is an inert substance that can cause beneficial and adverse reactions. Drugs can also—in addition to their real effects—produce placebo effects based on the health professional's attitudes and the patient's expectations.

Treatment Outcome

Treatment outcome can *never* be predicted with certainty for individual patients, and it depends on:

- The drug's physical and chemical properties (structure)—these are known and not variable factors
- The patient—most patients respond similarly to drugs, but differences in genetic backgrounds (e.g., family history), environment (e.g., air), habits (e.g., smoking, physical fitness), and compliance can cause unpredictable drug responses; these are variable factors
- The health professional—most health professionals are well trained, but differences exist in knowledge (relevant and irrelevant facts), experience, attitude (e.g., toward placebos) and instructions (written) provided; these are variable factors

Drug Use

Use of a particular drug is based on *benefit vs. risk*; the benefits of the use of a drug *must* outweigh risks to the patient.

Some abbreviations as found on drug prescriptions:

d:	day
q.:	every
q.4.h:	every 4 hours
q.d.:	every day
q.o.d.:	every other day
b.i.d.:	twice a day
t.i.d.:	three times a day
q.i.d.:	four times a day
t.i.w.:	three times a week
h.s.:	at bed time
p.c.:	after meals
ad lib., p.r.n.:	use when or as needed

Implications for the Physical Therapist

- Patients today are often afraid to take medications because of widely publicized adverse reactions. Advise patients that drugs are given only when the benefit outweighs the risk, and that drugs should be taken as recommended. Many adverse reactions are listed as possibilities for legal reasons, and their actual occurrence is often doubtful. Tell patients that taking a drug is like driving a car: There is a definite benefit involved, but there is always the possibility of an accident.

- Advise patients that many adverse reactions are minor and often disappear if the drug is discontinued early on. Patients should not "look" for adverse reactions but only be aware of such reactions when they occur, and that they should contact the physician immediately.

- Inform patients that humans are all individuals and that therapeutic and adverse reactions can vary from individual to individual. If no therapeutic effect is experienced or an adverse reaction manifests itself, patients should contact the physician.

- Inform patients that generic drugs can look different from brand name drugs but contain exactly the same active ingredients and are as effective as the brand name drug, with very few exceptions as indicated by the physician.

ACE Inhibitors

Common Drugs (selection of some of the most commonly used drugs)

Benazepril (Lotensin)
Captopril (Capoten)
Enalapril (Vasotec)
Fosinopril (Monopril)
Lisinopril (Prinivil, Zestril)
Moexipril (Univasc)
Perindopril (Aceon)
Quinapril (Accupril)
Ramipril (Altace)
Trandolapril (Mavik)

Indications

ACE inhibitors are indicated in:

- *Hypertension or elevated blood pressure*, which can have many causes and be treated in various ways. One is through the angiotensin system. The enzyme renin is released from the kidneys, which converts angiotensinogen into angiotensin I. The enzyme angiotension-converting enzyme (ACE) converts this to angiotension II. Angiotensin II acts on angiotension receptors in the blood vessels, causing vasoconstriction and increases in blood pressure. In addition, angiotension II increases aldosterone secretion, which leads to salt and water retention, adding to the increased pressure. Drugs inhibit the enzyme ACE, reduce formation of angiotensin II, reduce blood pressure, and can reduce the risk of secondary myocardial infarctions and strokes.

- *Congestive heart failure (CHF)*, where the heart cannot pump enough blood to other organs of the body. This results in an enlarged heart with the patient quickly becoming fatigued and short of breath (pulmonary edema) during even the slightest exertion. ACE inhibitors cause vasodilation, decrease afterload, and reduce peripheral resistance, which helps the heart to eject blood more easily and efficiently.

- Other uses include decreased progression of diabetic nephropathy, possibly by dilating renal blood vessels and increasing blood flow to the kidney (captopril); and treating migraine headaches (lisinopril) by an uncertain mechanism.

- Although all of these drugs are ACE inhibitors, their indications and dosages vary among patients and the diseases to be treated. Black patients with hypertension seem to respond less well to some of these drugs.

Examples of Common Dosages

(general guidelines, many different dosage schedules)

Benazepril: 5–40 mg 1–2 times daily PO

Captopril: 12.5–150 mg 3 times daily PO

Enalapril: 2.5–40 mg 1–2 times daily PO

Fosinopril: 10–80 mg once daily PO with a maximum of 80 mg/day

Lisinopril: 10–40 mg once daily PO

Moexipril: 7.5–30 mg once daily PO

Perindopril: 4–16 mg 1–2 times daily PO

Quinapril: 10–80 mg once daily PO

Ramipril: 2.5–20 mg/day in 1–2 divided doses PO

Trandolapril: 1–4 mg once daily PO

Administration

These drugs are given intravenously and by mouth. They vary in onset between 20 to 60 minutes and have a duration of action of 6 to 24 hours.

Contraindications

These drugs are contraindicated in cases of hypersensitivity, with some cross-sensitivity among the drugs. They should be used with caution in cases of renal or hepatic impairments. Mixing some ACE inhibitors with nonsteroidal antiinflammatory drugs (NSAIDs) can cause kidney failure.

Common Adverse Reactions

Adverse reactions include headache, dizziness, hypotension, cough, taste disturbances, and, rarely, agranulocytosis, neutropenia, or angioedema.

Drug Interactions

Hypotensive effects are enhanced by other antihypertensive drugs. Hyperkalemia may occur with potassium-sparing diuretics. Antacids may decrease absorption and effectiveness of ACE inhibitors. Sympathomimetic over-the-counter (OTC) cold medications can antagonize the blood-lowering effects of ACE inhibitors. ACE inhibitors can enhance the hypoglycemic action of hypoglycemics.

Implications for Physical Therapists

- Advise patients to change positions and get up slowly because orthostatic hypotension may occur, mostly in the beginning of therapy and in geriatric individuals. This can be aggravated if patients sweat heavily in a warm environment during strenuous exercise.

- If patients complain about a sore throat, notify or have patients notify the physician because this could be an early warning sign of agranulocytosis. If you notice or patients complain about swollen ankles or welts, notify or have patients contact the physician, because this could indicate an angioedema.

- Be careful when using a heated therapeutic pool because warm water can aggravate the vasodilatory effects of peripheral vascular dilators and lead to a marked decrease in blood pressure.

- Be aware that very young and older individuals might respond somewhat differently to medications. You will have to watch these patients more carefully because they often show more adverse reactions.

- Geriatric patients often receive multiple medications, sometimes prescribed by different physicians and obtained at different pharmacies. Inform patients to make a list of all medications and show this list to every physician. Also, patients should obtain all medications if possible from the same pharmacy because the same pharmacist could spot potentially dangerous drug interactions.

- Inform patient that therapeutic and adverse reactions can never be predicted with certainty because individuals will have different genetic and environmental backgrounds. It is mostly the patient who must monitor therapeutic progress and spot adverse reactions, but this can be helped by health professionals who can observe patients closely.

- Inform patients to take medications exactly as prescribed because inappropriate or missed doses can decrease the beneficial effects of a drug or increase its adverse reactions. The best way is to make a list and record the times when the drug should be taken.

- Inform patient that it is very important whether a drug should be taken with meals or before or after a meal because this can significantly affect the therapeutic response and adverse reactions.

- Inform patient that the drug should be taken as long as directed by a physician even if he or she feels better because, as in the case of antibiotics, remaining bacteria that do not cause clinical signs must still be eliminated.

- If a dose has been missed, inform the patient—unless otherwise instructed by the physician—to take the next dose if it is less than half the time before the next dose. For most drugs, the following is recommended: A drug should be taken every 6 hrs; if the last dose was taken at 8 am, the next doses should be taken at 2 pm and 8 pm. If the 2 pm dose was missed, it can still be taken at

4 pm but not at 6 pm; in this case it is better to skip the dose.

- Tell your patient that it is alright to split tablets because sometimes the higher dose costs the same as the lower dose. By receiving the higher dose and splitting, the patient can obtain double the lower doses for the same amount of money. Warn the patient that they should NOT split slow-release or extended tablets.

α Agonists

Common Drugs (selection of some of the most commonly used drugs)

Direct-acting α_1 agonists
Epinephrine (also beta activity) (Adrenalin, Ana-Guard, Primatene Mist, other)
Midodrine (ProAmatine)
Phenylephrine (Neo-Synephrine [OTC])
Direct-acting α_2 agonists (see Miscellaneous Vasodilators)
Clonidine (Catapres, Duraclon)
Direct/indirect-acting α agonists (also beta activity)
Ephedrine (generic)
Pseudoephedrine (Sudafed, Drixoral, Decofed, other [OTC])

Indications

α agonists are indicated in:

- *Nasal congestion* due to viral or allergic causes, which produces vasodilation and leakage of water in adjacent tissues. α1 and indirect-acting drugs constrict blood vessels, stop leakage, and open airways; common nasal sprays contain naphazoline, xylometazoline, phenylephrine, or oxymetazoline.
- *Allergic conditions* where part of the problem is vasodilation. α1 agonists and indirect-acting drugs constrict blood vessels. Ocular drugs to counteract congestion and redness are naphazoline, oxymetazoline, tetrahydrozoline, and phenylephrine. In case of an anaphylactic reaction, epinephrine subcutaneously (SC) is necessary.
- *Shock* caused by fluid loss, bleeding, or other causes. Drugs increase blood pressure by vasoconstriction, and cardiac stimulation in the case of indirect-acting drugs. Ephedrine is also used in cases of hypotension.
- *Bronchoconstriction*, where constriction of the bronchi interferes with airflow. Indirect-acting drugs and epinephrine (via action on beta receptors) are used as sprays or orally to open airways.
- *Ocular eye examinations*, where phenylephrine causes mydriasis, allowing better examination of the posterior parts of the eye.

Examples of Common Dosages
(general guidelines, many different dosage schedules)

Epinephrine: 0.1–0.5 mg to be repeated every 20 min–4 hr for asthma SC
Midodrine: 2.5–10 mg 2–3 times daily by mouth (PO)

Pseudoephedrine: 60 mg every
6 hr (not to exceed 240 mg/day)
Ephedrine: 25 mg 4 times a day PO

Administration

These drugs can be given SC, intramuscular (IM), IV, PO, via inhalation, and topical in the eye.

Contraindications

These drugs are contraindicated (or should be used with caution) in hypertension, arrhythmias, and prostatic hyperplasia (leading to urinary hesitancy and retention).

Common Adverse Reactions

- Adverse reactions include nervousness, restlessness, tremor, hypertension, angina, bradycardia (because of increased blood pressure), and arrhythmias. Indirect-acting drugs may cause central nervous system stimulation and anorexia.
- Nasal and ocular applications in rapid succession (after 2 to 3 days) can lead to a rebound effect in which congestion becomes worse with each application.
- For epinephrine only: Excessive use of inhalers can lead to bronchospasm.

Drug Interactions

- Drugs antagonize the effects of α blockers and antihypertensive drugs. They can precipitate a hypertensive crisis in conjunction with MAO inhibitors. Antacids that alkalinize the urine can intensify their effects.
- Foods that acidify (cheeses, fish, meat) or alkalinize (most fruits and vegetables) the urine can decrease or intensify effects.

Implications for Physical Therapists

- Some of these drugs are available OTC in nasal sprays, cold medications, and ocular solutions. Patients often assume that OTC drugs are safe and can be used without any precautions. Advise patients that they are still drugs and must be used with care and according to instructions.
- If you notice that blood pressure has increased in patients taking antihypertensive medication, or if patients show increased restlessness, inquire about the use of OTC medications. If an α agonist is being used, advise the patient to contact a physician.
- If you notice that your patients use nasal sprays too often, inform patients that they might suffer from a rebound effect and should contact a physician.
- Advise older men with benign prostatic hyperplasia that use of α agonists can lead to urinary hesitancy or even retention.

α Antagonists or Blockers

Common Drugs (selection of some of the most commonly used drugs)

Doxazosin (Cardura)
Phenoxybenzamine (Dibenzyline)
Prazosin (Minipress)
Tamsulosin (Flomax)
Terazosin (Hytrin)

Indications

α antagonists are indicated in:

- *Hypertension*, when vasoconstriction or increased peripheral resistance is a major cause of increased blood pressure. α blockers block α receptors, relax blood vessels, decrease peripheral resistance, and lower blood pressure.
- *Benign prostatic hyperplasia*, in which α blockers relax the sphincter muscle, leading to more efficient bladder emptying, and relax the capsule/muscles of the prostate, providing improved urinary flow.

Examples of Common Dosages

(general guidelines, many different dosage schedules)

Doxazosin: 1–16 mg once daily PO
Phenoxybenzamine: 10–40 mg twice daily PO
Prazosin: 1–15 mg 2–3 times daily PO (not to exceed 40 mg/day)
Tamsulosin: 0.4–0.8 mg once daily
Terazosin: 1–5 mg once or twice a day PO (not to exceed 20 mg/day)

Administration

These drugs are administered PO. Some, such as phentolamine, are only given IV or IM.

Contraindications

These drugs are contraindicated (or should be used with caution) in patients with hypersensitivity to these drugs or low blood pressure.

Common Adverse Reactions

Common adverse reactions include headache, stuffy nose, fatigue, palpitations, tachycardia (as blood pressure drops, heart rate increases reflexively), marked "first dose" (syncope), and later on, less severe orthostatic hypotension. Geriatric patients are at increased risk of experiencing adverse reactions.

Drug Interactions

There is an increased risk of hypotension with drugs that also lower blood pressure, including alcohol, sildenafil, and others. Some cold medications containing phenylephrine or other α-agonistic compounds can antagonize actions of α blockers.

Implications for Physical Therapists

- Be careful when patients change positions or stand up, because of possible orthostatic hypotension, particularly at the beginning of therapy or in geriatric patients.
- Watch patients when they stop after strenuous exercise because risk of a hypotensive episode is increased.
- Be careful when using a heated therapeutic pool because warm water can aggravate the vasodilatory effects of peripheral vascular dilators and lead to a marked decrease in blood pressure.

Alternative Medications

Introduction

Alternative medications include all herbal preparations, vitamins, minerals, and other products used for other than nutritional reasons, but not prescription drugs and over-the-counter (OTC) medications.

Prescription and OTC drugs have to be approved by the FDA after companies have performed extensive studies in animals and humans to establish efficacy and toxicity. Drugs are then approved for specific indications and must state active ingredient(s), inactive ingredients, exact dose, and administration schedule, as well as suggested mode of action and adverse reactions as compiled, e.g., in the *Physicians' Desk Reference* (PDR).

Alternative medications are handled like food by the FDA and must state content but not dose. Companies are not required to submit proof of efficacy and toxicity as long as they do not make a specific health claim, but remain vague in their indications. Because of this lack of control, products can contain varying amounts of the specified item and sometimes are subject to fraudulent practices.

Claims for their beneficial effects are often based on historical aspects ("has been used by the Chinese for centuries"), folklore ("this herb has been known for centuries to help people sleep"), and some epidemiological correlations ("a survey of a large number of individuals has shown that individuals who consume a lot of a specific mineral will have less breast cancer"—although this is a valid correlation, it does not indicate that this mineral indeed prevents this cancer). In addition, there is the misconception by many people that naturally occurring alternative medications are safe because they are derived from nature—this is wrong because natural products can be quite toxic (e.g., poison ivy, poisonous mushrooms).

At present, a number of controlled clinical trials are being conducted with certain alternative medications, and in the years to come more information about the benefits and risks of alternative medications will become more evident. At present, many hopes about these medications have been disproven by clinical trials. Thus, most information available today is tentative at best and is constantly changing.

Vitamins

Vitamins are a group of unrelated substances essential for many normal biochemical and physiological processes (e.g., catalysts for enzymes), which are obtained from the diet or synthesized (e.g., vitamin D) by the body. For nutritional purposes, they are required only in small quantities as estimated by the Recommended Dietary Allowances (RDA) and are present in sufficient amounts in a balanced daily diet (meats, carbohydrates, dairy products, and a lot of fruits and vegetables—many foods are also now vitamin fortified) to prevent vitamin deficiency diseases. There is no need for supplementation to maintain a healthy body and mind in healthy individuals eating a balanced diet, except perhaps for some infants and older people. Those with work-related conditions; heavily menstruating, pregnant, or lactating women; individuals consuming improper diets; those with certain diseases; and those on some drug therapies may benefit from supplementation.

Recently, higher doses of certain vitamins have been suggested to prevent or to cure certain diseases, such as emphysema, asthma, and bronchitis; cardiovascular diseases; cancer; aging; mental disorders; the common cold; and other health problems. At present, there is no firm evidence that this is indeed the case. However, very high doses of some vitamins (e.g., vitamins A, D, and perhaps E) can be quite toxic and/or increase the risk of certain diseases for which they were actually recommended in the first place. Legitimate and documented uses of vitamin preparations as preventive or curative measures include those that slow down age-related macular degeneration (vitamins E, C, and beta carotene) and that increase calcium absorption (vitamin D). If vitamins are used, preparations that carry the label of the United States Pharmacopeia are recommended. This private organization, recognized by Congress, has established some standards for vitamins and minerals (e.g., strength or amount of active ingredient; purity; disintegration; dissolution).

Minerals

Minerals are necessary for many biochemical processes (e.g., co-factors for enzymes), physiological functions (e.g., hemoglobin), and structural requirements (e.g., teeth, bones). Optimal mineral intake values for humans are still estimates, but a balanced diet seems to provide all necessary minerals to healthy individuals. In addition, many foods are supplemented with minerals.

Higher doses of minerals have also been suggested for healthy individuals to prevent or cure health problems. No firm evidence supports the use of minerals, with the exception of iron (under supervision of a physician because it can be toxic in high amounts), calcium (with vitamin D) to increase bone formation, and zinc for retardation of age-related macular degeneration (on advice of an ophthalmologist).

Herbal Preparations

A variety of available herbal medications claim or suggest many benefits, most of which are not medically verified or have been proven wrong. Some of these preparations have also been found to cause significant health problems or even death (such as ephedra) or can significantly interfere with prescription drugs, either reducing the drugs' efficacy or increasing their toxicity.

Ginger may reduce nausea and vomiting—there's some evidence—

and valerian may treat anxiety and insomnia, and indeed has some calming properties. However, it has also been claimed, for example, that echinacea stimulates the immune system; if true, then it would be strongly contraindicated in cases of autoimmune diseases. Garlic is supposed to reduce the risk of cardiovascular disease, but bleeding episodes can occur with heparin, warfarin, and aspirin. Gingko biloba may increase memory and cognition, and improve circulation, although it too can interfere with heparin, warfarin, and aspirin. St. John's wort may improve mood, and there is some support for its effects on mild depression, but it can interfere with some antiviral and anticancer medications.

Biochemicals

A number of biochemicals are offered for a variety of health problems, most of which have again not been documented through scientific trials.

For instance, melatonin is a naturally occurring substance in our body that physiologically is involved in sleep and that is now marketed as a sleep promoter. Although its use is safe, it does not seem to induce sleep and help jet lag, except in some individuals. Glucosamine and chondroitin are components needed to build and maintain articular cartilage and synovial fluid. It has been claimed that their use can help patients with osteoarthritis, but although some individuals indeed seem to benefit,

most individuals do not seem to get relief. Unfortunately, both compounds can cause significant gastrointestinal (GI) problems such as nausea, cramping, and heart burn. Omega-3 polyunsaturated fatty acids might be beneficial to prevent certain cardiovascular risks, but many experts advise obtaining these biochemicals from eating fish 2–3 times a week.

Implications for the Physical Therapist

- It is important to stress to patients that the most important aspects of maintaining good health and preventing diseases are a well-balanced diet, an optimistic outlook in life, and daily physical exercise.
- It is important to inform patients that the benefits of alternative medications with exceptions as outlined before are still unproven, that use of these preparations is not risk free, and that some of them can interfere detrimentally with prescription drugs. They should not be taken without the advice of a physician, and their use must be stated when a medical history is taken.
- It is important to inform patients that it is better to spend available money on good food and not on alternative medications.
- It is important to warn the patient about advertisements of these products on TV, in newspapers, or on websites. When searching the Internet, attention should be paid to websites that

end in .edu or .gov, because these derive from universities and government agencies and may have more research behind what they state. Many other websites might or might not be correct, and the intention of many is mostly to sell but not to inform.

Angiotensin II Receptor Antagonists

Common Drugs (selection of some of the most commonly used drugs)

Candesartan (Atacand)
Eprosartan (Teveten)
Irbesartan (Avapro)
Losartan (Cozaar)
Olmesartan (Benicar)
Telmisartan (Micardis)
Valsartan (Diovan)

Indications

Angiotensin II receptor antagonists are indicated in:

- *Hypertension*, left untreated is linked to myocardial infarctions and strokes. These antagonists block the action of the vasoconstrictor angiotensin II on its receptor and also reduce the secretion of aldosterone. Both actions lower blood pressure and can reduce the risk of secondary myocardial infarctions and strokes.
- *Congestive heart failure*, (CHF) when the heart cannot pump enough blood to other organs of the body. This results in an enlarged heart, with the patient quickly becoming fatigued and short of breath (pulmonary edema) during even the slightest exertion. These drugs (especially candesartan, valsartan) cause vasodilatation, reduce after load, and reduce peripheral resistance, which helps the heart to eject blood more easily and efficiently.

- Other uses include *diabetic nephropathy* in type II diabetes, possibly by dilating renal blood vessels and increasing blood flow to the kidney (irbesartan, losartan).
- While all of these drugs block angiotensin II receptors, their indications and dosages vary among patients and the diseases to be treated. Black patients with hypertension seem to respond less well to some of these drugs.

Examples of Common Dosages
(general guidelines, many different dosage schedules)

Candesartan: 2–32 mg once or twice daily PO
Eprosartan: 400–800 mg once daily PO
Irbesartan: 150–300 mg once daily PO
Losartan: 25–100 mg once daily PO
Olmesartan: 10–20 mg once daily PO
Telmisartan: 20–80 mg once daily PO
Valsartan: 40–320 once or twice daily PO

Administration

These drugs are given mostly PO and often used in combination with other antihypertensive medications.

Contraindications

These drugs are contraindicated (or should be used with caution) in patients with renal and hepatic impairments, and certain cardiac conditions.

Common Adverse Reactions

Adverse reactions include dizziness, fatigue, hypotension, angioedema, and in rare cases, renal failure.

Drug Interactions

- NSAIDS may decrease the effectiveness of these drugs. They can aggravate potassium retention when using potassium-sparing diuretics, and enhance the effects of other antihypertensive drugs.
- Effects are increased with mistletoe, astragalus, black cohosh, and others.

Implications for Physical Therapists

- Advise patients to change positions and get up slowly because orthostatic hypotension may occur, mostly in the beginning of therapy and in geriatric individuals. This can be aggravated if patients sweat heavily in a warm environment during strenuous exercise.
- Be careful when using a heated therapeutic pool, because warm water can aggravate the vasodilatory effects of peripheral vascular dilators and lead to a marked decrease in blood pressure.

Antiarrhythmics

Common Drugs (selection of some of the most commonly used drugs)

Class IA
  Disopyramide (Norpace)
  Procainamide (Procanbid, Promine, Pronestyl)
  Quinidine (Quinalan, Cardioquin, Quinora, other)
Class IB
  Lidocaine (Xylocaine, other)
  Mexiletine (Mexitil)
  Phenytoin (Dilantin, Phenytex)
  Tocainide (Tonocard)
Class IC
  Flecainide (Tambocor)
  Propafenone (Rythmol)
Class II or β blockers (see β Antagonists or Blockers)
  Acebutolol

  Esmolol
  Propranolol
  Sotalol
Class III
  Amiodarone (Cordarone, Pacerone)
  Ibutilide (Corvert)
Class IV or calcium channel blockers (see Calcium Channel Blockers)
  Verapamil
  Miscellaneous drugs
  Adenosine
  Atropine (see *Anticholinergics*)

Indications

Antiarrhythmic drugs are indicated in:

- *Arrhythmias* (better called dysrhythmias as arrhythmia means "no rhythm"), which are caused by malfunctioning pacemaker cells unable to maintain normal activity; emergence of new pacemaker cells competing with the original ones; interruption of normal conductance over the heart in that conduction can not reach certain areas (heart blocks) or in an upward and circular fashion with reexcitation of cardiac tissue (reentry); or a combination of these causes. There are several different types of arrhythmias, which can range from harmless to life-threatening.

- These abnormalities are specifically influenced by the different drug classes, which try to normalize conduction patterns by selectively affecting β receptors or individual electrolyte fluxes (sodium, potassium, or calcium), and reestablish a normal rhythm. Generally, class I drugs block sodium channels and are used for ventricular dysrhythmias, such as ventricular ectopic beats (skipped heartbeats) and ventricular tachycardias. Quinidine can be used for atrial tachycardias as well. Class II drugs are β blockers and are used for sinus tachycardia, atrial fibrillation and flutter, and some ventricular dysrhythmias. Class III drugs slow potassium effluxes and are used mostly for ventricular dysrhythmias, but can also be used for atrial fibrillation. Class IV drugs are calcium channel blockers and are used in atrial fibrillation and flutter, and supraventricular tachycardia. Miscellaneous drugs such as adenosine are used mostly for diagnostic purposes, and atropine is used for certain bradycardias.

Examples of Common Dosages
(general guidelines, many different dosage schedules)

Disopyramide: 100–200 mg every 6 hr PO or 200–400 mg every 12 hr PO for slow release preparations

Procainamide: 1 g followed by 50 mg/kg/day every 6 hr PO

Quinidine: 200–600 mg every 2–3 hr up to 4 g/day

Lidocaine injections: infusions at various dosages

Mexiletine: 200–400 mg followed by 200–400 mg every 8 hr PO

Phenytoin: 1 g divided over one day then 500 mg/day for 2 days PO

Tocainide: 400–1800 mg/day in divided doses PO

Flecainide: 50 mg every 6–12 hr up to 300 mg/day PO

Propafenone: 150 mg every 8 hr up to 900 mg/day PO

Amiodarone: 800–160 mg/day for 1–3 weeks, followed by 600–800 mg for 1 month, and followed by 400 mg/day PO

Ibutilide: IV infusions at different rates

Verapamil: 240–320 mg/day in 3–4 divided doses PO

Adenosine: IV infusions at different rates

Atropine: IV bolus injections at different dosages

Administration

These drugs can be given IV (bolus, infusion) and PO. It is important to follow exactly the prescribed dosage protocol as these drugs can be quite toxic if taken too frequently or at higher-than-prescribed dosages.

Contraindications

These drugs are contraindicated (or should be used with care) in patients with heart failure, myocardial ischemia, and previous myocardial infarctions.

Common Adverse Reactions

These drugs carry a high risk of adverse reactions. Most drugs have the potential to normalize one type of dysrhythmia while causing another type. They can cause dizziness, confusion, and nausea, which are sometimes indications of the presence of such a dysrhythmia. Depending on the class, Class I drugs can cause hypotension, bradycardia, edema, syncope (fainting), heart failure, leucopenia, constipation, urinary retention, and, rarely, agranulocytosis. In addition, tinnitus (ringing in the ears) and hearing loss occur mostly with quinidine; GI bleeding with mexiletine; nephritis (urine discoloration) and Stevens-Johnson syndrome with phenytoin; and respiratory depression with flecainide. Class II drugs can cause bronchoconstriction and excessive bradycardia. Class III drugs are relatively safe except for amiodarone, which can cause deposits in the cornea, a toxic epidermal necrolysis, and pulmonary fibrosis (warning signals are dyspnea, cough, and pain). Class IV drugs or calcium channel blockers may cause bradycardia and hypotension.

Drug Interactions

- These drugs can interact with other antidysrhythmic drugs, β blockers, anticholinergics, and other drugs.
- Toxicity is increased by a large number of herbal products. Alcohol and caffeine-containing foods and drinks can aggravate dysrhythmias.

Implications for Physical Therapists

- Advise patients that these are very effective but also potentially dangerous drugs and that patients must adhere strictly to the prescribed dosing schedule, because deviations can significantly reduce therapeutic and increase toxic effects.
- Advise patients to adhere strictly to office appointments and lab tests because early recognition of an adverse reaction through such lab tests can detect and prevent subsequent health problems.
- If you notice peripheral edema, or patients complain about dyspnea, notify or have patients contact a physician because dosage adjustments or a different drug might be indicated.
- Have patients change position slowly, particularly during early therapy when dizziness and orthostatic hypotension might occur, causing patients to fall.
- If patients complain about nausea and dizziness, have them contact

their physician. These symptoms could be a warning signal of another dysrhythmia.

- Advise patients to abstain from caffeine-containing drinks or foods, as they can aggravate dysrhythmias.
- If a patient on quinidine complains about tinnitus, have the patient contact a physician, because quinidine use can lead to hearing problems.

- If patients complain about a fever followed by a rash and painful skin areas, have them immediately call a physician. This could be a warning signal for a toxic epidermal necrolysis, which could be very serious.
- Check pulse rate during more strenuous exercises or if patient becomes prematurely fatigued and stop exercises if abnormal rate is felt.

Antiasthmatics

Common Drugs (selection of some of the most commonly used drugs)

β Agonists (see β Agonists)
    Albuterol
    Formoterol
    Bitolterol
    Levalbuterol
    Metaproterenol
    Pirbuterol
    Terbutaline
Anticholinergics (see
    Anticholinergics)
    Ipratropium
    Tiotropium
Adrenergics (see α Agonists)
    Epinephrine
Corticosteroids (see
    Corticosteroids)
    Beclomethasone
    Betamethasone
    Budesonide
    Cortisone
    Dexamethasone
    Flunisolide
    Fluticasone
    Hydrocortisone
    Methylprednisolone
    Prednisone
    Triamcinolone

Leukotriene antagonists
    Zafirlukast (Accolate)
Mast cell stabilizer (see
    Antihistamines)
    Cromolyn
    Nedocromil
Phosphodiesterase inhibitors
    Theophylline (Accurbron,
        Bronkodyl, Lanophyllin,
        other)
Monoclonal antibodies (see
    Antihistamines)
    Omalizumab

Indications

Antiasthmatics are indicated in:

- Asthma, which is caused by bronchoconstriction (constricting action of histamine, leukotrienes, and acetylcholine) and inflammation. Both narrow the bronchi and cause "air hunger" (wheezing). Drugs relax the bronchi by blocking the constricting causes (anticholinergic drugs, leukotriene antagonists, histamine antagonists or reducers) or by promoting relaxation (β agonists, theophylline), as well as reducing inflammation (corticosteroids). In all cases, the inner diameter of the bronchi is increased and a more efficient airflow is established.

- Other conditions such as chronic obstructive pulmonary disease (COPD) and emphysema, two lung diseases in which the lung is damaged (for example, by smoking), making it difficult to breathe.

Examples of Common Dosages
(general guidelines, many different dosage schedules)

Theophylline: 100–800 mg every 6 hr PO

Zafirlukast: 20 mg b.i.d. PO

Administration

These drugs can be given IV, SC, or PO. Onset of action is fastest with inhaled preparations and adverse reactions are less severe.

Contraindications

Theophylline should not be used in patients with tachydysrhythmias.

Common Adverse Reactions

Adverse reactions for leukotriene antagonists include headache, nausea, dyspepsia, and the very rare but potentially dangerous Churg-Strauss syndrome. Theophylline can cause restlessness, insomnia, seizures, tachycardia, dysrhythmias, and dyspepsia.

Drug Interactions

Interleukin antagonists interact with a small number of drugs such as aspirin and warfarin. Theophylline increases the cardiotoxicity of β blockers. Toxicity of theophylline is increased by both black and green teas, coffee, and ephedra.

Implications for Physical Therapists

- If a patient on zafirlukast complains about a rash and nodules, inform or have the patient contact a physician immediately, because this could be the beginning of Churg-Strauss syndrome.
- Advise patients taking theophylline to take the medication exactly as prescribed, because the dosage schedule is very important and deviations can increase the risk of adverse effects (the margin of safety is very small).

Antibacterials

Common Drugs (selection of some of the most commonly used drugs)

Penicillins
  Amoxicillin (Augmentin [with clavulanate])
  Penicillin G (Bicillin, Megacillin)

Other
Cephalosporins
  Cefazolin (Ancef)
  Cefepime (Maxipime)
  Cefotaxime (Claforan)
  Cephalexin (Keflex)
  Other

Quinolones
  Ciprofloxacin (Cipro, ProQuin)
  Levofloxacin (Levaquin)
  Other
Aminoglycosides
  Gentamicin (Garamycin)
  Other
Tetracyclines
  Tetracycline (Tetracyn,
    Achromycin, other)
  Other
Macrolides
  Azithromycin (Zithromax,
    Zmax)
  Other
Sulfonamides
  Sulfisoxazole (Gantrisin)
  Trimethoprim (Primsol,
    Trimpex, other)
  Other
Miscellaneous Drugs
  Bacitracin
  Imipenem (Primaxin [with
    cilastatin])

Indications

Antibacterial drugs are indicated in:

- *Bacterial infections*, in which drugs are specific for a particular bacterial species or strain. Drugs act mostly through the following mechanisms:
  - Inhibition of synthesis and/or damage to the peptidoglycan component of the bacterial cell wall. This biochemical is unique and necessary to the microbial cell wall, and its disruption kills the microorganism (e.g., penicillins, cephalosporins, imipenem, and other).
  - Inhibition of synthesis and/or damage to the microbial cytoplasmic membrane (e.g., polymyxins).
- Modification of synthesis and/or metabolism of microbial nucleic acids by affecting two microbial enzymes, gyrase and topoisomerase, which are necessary for replication and cell division (e.g., quinolones).
- Inhibition or modification of microbial protein synthesis by disrupting microbial ribosomal function and impairing protein synthesis (e.g., aminoglycosides, tetracyclines, macrolides).
- Inhibition or modification of microbial cell metabolism by affecting folic acid synthesis/metabolism, which has to be synthesized by bacteria and which is necessary for their nucleic acid synthesis (e.g., sulfonamides, trimethoprim).

Examples are ciprofloxacin and imipenem for *Bacillus anthracis* (anthrax); penicillin G for *Clostridium tetani* (tetanus); amoxicillin or trimethoprim/sulfonamide for *Escherichia coli* (bacteremia, urinary tract infections); cefotaxime for *Haemophilus influenzae* (otitis, pneumonia); penicillin G for *Streptococcus* (endocarditis); cefotaxime and ciprofloxacin for *Salmonella typhi* (typhoid fever); and cephalosporins or aminoglycoside for *Klebsiella pneumoniae* (pneumonia).

Examples of Common Dosages
(general guidelines, many different dosage schedules)

Amoxicillin: 750–1750 mg in divided doses daily PO

Penicillin G: 2.4 million units IM

Cefazolin: 250–2000 mg every 6–8 hrs IM, IV

Cefepime: 0.5–2000 mg every 12 hrs IV, IM

Cefotaxime: 1–2 g every 4–12 hrs IM, IV

Cephalexin: 250–1000 mg every 6 hrs PO

Ciprofloxacin: 100–500 mg every 12 hrs daily PO

Levofloxacin: 250–750 mg daily PO, IV

Gentamicin: 3–6 mg/kg/day in divided doses every 8 hrs IV INF, or 3 mg/kg/day in divided doses every 8 hrs IM

Tetracycline: 250–500 mg every 6 hrs daily PO

Azithromycin: 250–2000 mg daily PO

Sulfisoxazole: 2–4 g followed by 1–2 g daily PO

Trimethoprim: 100 mg every 12 hrs daily PO

Imipenem: 250–1000 mg every 6–8 hrs IV

Administration

Depending on the drug, they are administered PO, IV, or IM.

Contraindications

These drugs are contraindicated (or should be used with caution) in patients with renal and/or hepatic problems.

Common Adverse Reactions

In general, antibacterial drugs can cause nausea, vomiting, allergic reactions, pseudomembranous colitis, Stevens-Johnson syndrome, and superinfections. In addition, penicillins and cephalosporins are relatively free of adverse reactions except allergic reactions, with some cross-sensitivity between classes. Similarly, macrolides show mostly allergic reactions. Aminoglycosides are more toxic and might cause nephro- and ototoxicity. Tetracyclines cause photosensitivity to UV light and should not be given to growing individuals, because they can stain teeth and interfere with bone calcification. Quinolones can cause visual disturbances, photosensitization, and inflammations of the tendons. Sulfonamides taken at high doses may cause renal stone formation and necessitate the consumption of large amounts of fluids.

Drug Interactions

- A large number of interactions exist. Penicillins can decrease the effects of contraceptives. Tetracyclines can reduce the efficacy of penicillins. Some cephalosporins show increased toxicity with a large number of herbal preparations.
- Generally, acidophilus should not be used with antiinfectives. Antacids and/or dairy products (calcium and other metals) decrease efficacy of tetracyclines, macrolides, and quinolones.

Implications for Physical Therapists

- Advise patients to follow the prescription schedule strictly and to continue taking drugs even if clinical signs or symptoms have subsided. The schedule is designed to eradicate the microorganism at all sites in the body, even those where no clinical problems are manifested.

- If patients exhibit an unexplained rash, inform or have them contact a physician, because this could be the beginning of Stevens-Johnson syndrome.
- If patients have abdominal discomfort, ask them to check their stool. If pus or mucus is detected, contact or ask patients to contact a physician because this could be a sign of pseudomembranous colitis.
- Advise patients and reinforce the warning that tetracyclines and quinolones must be taken as prescribed, because food or antacids can render them ineffective.
- Patients taking quinolones complaining about tendon pain, particularly pain of the Achilles tendon, should not be exercised strenuously. They should be carefully evaluated and the physician informed. This could indicate tendonitis, possibly requiring a change in medication.
- Avoid UV light therapy, or cover unexposed areas well, of patients on tetracyclines and quinolones. These drugs can cause photosensitization.

Anticholinergics

Common Drugs (selection of some of the most commonly used drugs)

Atropine (generic and in belladonna)
Dicyclomine (Bentyl)
Hyoscyamine (Levsin, Anaspaz, Donnamar, other)
Ipratropium (Atrovent, other)
Oxybutynin (Ditropan)
Scopolamine (Transderm-Scop)
Tiotropium (Spiriva)
Tolterodine (Detrol)

Benztropine (Cogentin)
Biperiden (Akineton)
Trihexyphenidyl (Artane)

Indications

Anticholinergics are indicated in:

- *Arrhythmias* such as sinus bradycardia, where they block cardiac muscarinic receptors, increase heart rate and normalize cardiac rhythm.
- *Peptic ulcer and irritable bowel syndrome*, in which they antagonize excessive muscarinic receptor stimulation, and gastric and intestinal activity.
- *Urinary bladder hypermotility including enuresis*, where they block muscarinic receptors, relax the bladder and decrease frequent urination or bed wetting.
- *Asthma*, where they block bronchial muscarinic receptors, reduce secretion into and dilate the bronchi with increased air flow.
- *Cases of pesticide/nerve gas poisoning*, in which they protect the muscarinic receptors from excessive acetylcholine stimulation caused by inhibition of acetylcholinesterase by these agents.
- *Ocular applications*, where they block muscarinic receptors dilate the pupil and relax the ciliary body (topically applied tropi-

camide, cyclopentolate, and atropine).

The drugs under the line are used in the therapy of:

- *Parkinson disease*, which is a movement disorder characterized by a mask-like face, shuffling gait, and pill-rolling tremor. The cause is believed to be—among other problems—an overactivity of cholinergic and underactivity of dopaminergic activity in the basal ganglia of the brain. These drugs reduce cholinergic overactivity and restore the balance between the two systems, improving rigidity and tremor.

Examples of Common Dosages
(general guidelines, many different dosage schedules)

Atropine: Various schedules, mostly as given as belladonna extract 10–100 mg PO (calculated as 0.5 mg alkaloid).

Dicyclomine: 10–20 mg 3–4 times daily PO (up to 160 mg/day)

Hyoscyamine: 0.125–0.25 mg 3–4 times daily PO, or 0.375–0.75 mg every 12 hrs as sustained release form PO

Ipratropium: 1–4 inhalations 3–4 times daily

Oxybutynin: 5 mg 2–3 times daily PO, or 5–10 mg PO once daily as sustained release form

Tiotropium: Inhalation of 18 mcg once daily

Benztropin: 1 to 2 mg/day in 1–2 divided doses PO (up to 6 mg/day)

Biperidin: 2 mg 1–4 times daily PO (not to exceed 16 mg/day)

Trihexyphenidyl: 1–6 mg/day in divided doses PO

Administration
These drugs can be given IV, IM, inhalation, and PO.

Contraindications
These drugs are contraindicated (or should be used with caution) in patients with cardiovascular problems, seizure disorders, prostatic hyperplasia, and GI hypomotility.

Common Adverse Reactions
Adverse reactions include confusion (more severe in geriatric patients), dry skin and mouth, decreased sweating, blurred vision, constipation, and urinary hesitancy and retention (mainly in geriatric patients). They may cause contact lens intolerance because of dry eye.

Drug Interactions
- These drugs can slow the absorption of a number of other drugs and can antagonize the effects of some antiglaucoma medications.
- Increased anticholinergic effects have been reported with jimson weed, Scopolia, and angel's trumpet.

Addendum
In addition, there are a number of antihistamines, antipsychotics, and antidepressants that show strong anticholinergic effects (see *Anticholinergics*).

Implications for Physical Therapists
- Expect some increases in heart rate because of blockade of cardiac muscarinic receptors.

- Expect some mental confusion in older patients taking anticholinergic drugs (or drugs that have anticholinergic properties).
- When exercising a patient on anticholinergic medication, keep the environment cool because there is the risk of heat prostration caused by decreased ability to sweat and lose heat.

Anticonvulsants

Common Drugs (selection of some of the most commonly used drugs)
Barbiturates
    Phenobarbital (Luminal, Solfoton, other)
    Primidone (Mysoline)
    Other
Benzodiazepines
    Clonazepam (Klonopin)
    Diazepam (Valium)
    Other
Hydantoins
    Phenytoin (Dilantin, Phenytex)
    Other
Succinimides
    Ethosuximide (Zarontin)
    Other
Carboxylic acids
    Valproic acid (Depakene, Depacon, other)
Iminostilbenes
    Carbamazepine (Tegretol, Atretol, other)
    Oxcarbazepine (Trileptal)
Second generation drugs
    Gabapentin (Neurontin)
    Lamotrigine (Lamictal)
    Tiagabine (Gabitril)
    Other

Indications

Anticonvulsants are indicated in:
- *Epilepsy*, characterized by seizures that are episodes of sudden and uncontrolled but transient hyperexcitability of small groups of neurons or "foci." The cause for that sudden hyperexcitability or spontaneous but unnecessary neuronal overactivity are poorly understood, but defects in the GABA system of the brain, excessive $Na+$ fluxes, and faulty $K+$ and $Ca++$ fluxes have been suggested. These discharges can produce muscle contractions (convulsions) or behavioral abnormality (loss of consciousness). They can be localized or spread over the entire brain and can be divided into partial and generalized seizures. Anticonvulsants prevent this unwanted and deleterious hyperexcitability of certain brain areas or to reduce it to initiate or to reduce it to a nonpathological level. Most drugs increase the action of the inhibitory neurotransmitter GABA, which opens chloride channels, causes hyperpolarization, and slows neuronal firing. Phenytoin blocks sodium channels, which slows the influx of sodium and prevents or reduces depolarization. Valproic acid affects potassium channels, leading to hyperpolarization and, again, a

reduction in neuronal firing. The mechanism of the other drugs is still quite unknown. In addition to these mechanisms, other neuronal effects play supporting or even crucial roles.

- Other uses for some selective drugs include essential tremors, restless leg syndrome, panic disorders, neuropathic pain, certain dysrhythmias, manic episodes, and trigeminal neuralgia.

Examples of Common Dosages
(general guidelines, many different dosage schedules)

Phenobarbital: 1–3 mg/kg/day in divided doses or total dose at bedtime PO

Primidone: 100–250 mg 3–4 times daily up to 2 g/day PO

Clonazepam: 1.5 mg/day in 3 divided doses up to 20 mg/day PO

Diazepam: 2–10 mg 3–4 times daily, or 15–30 mg once daily for extended release preparations, PO

Phenytoin: 1 g as loading dose in 3–4 divided doses and later as maintenance dose 300–600 mg/day PO

Ethosuximide: 250–750 daily PO

Valproic acid: 10–15 mg/kg/day in 2–3 divided doses, not to exceed 60 mg/kg/day PO

Carbamazepine: 200 mg 2 times daily up to 800–1600 mg/day PO

Oxcarbazepine: 300–600 mg 2 times daily PO

Gabapentin: 900–1800 mg/day in 1–3 divided doses PO

Lamotrigine: 50–500 mg/day in 2 divided doses PO

Tiagabine: 4 mg/day in divided doses up to 56 mg/day PO

Administration
Most drugs are given PO, but for certain conditions they have to be injected or infused. Drugs are often prescribed in combination. Drugs must be taken at precise dosages and schedules to be maximally effective.

Contraindications
Drugs should not be used or must be used with caution in patients with renal and hepatic diseases.

Common Adverse Reactions
All drugs will cause, to a varying degree, of gastric discomfort, sedation, drowsiness, and ataxia (confusion occurs mostly in geriatric patients). Barbiturates may cause paradoxical excitement in selected individuals. Some drugs such as barbiturates, oxcarbazine, gabapentin, and lamotrigine can cause Stevens-Johnson syndrome. Other drugs such as barbiturates and carbamazepine can cause blood disorders (agranulocytosis, leucopenia, megaloplastic or aplastic anemia). Phenytoin is associated with gingival hyperplasia, hirsutism, nephritis (colored urine), and hepatitis. Valproic acid may cause hepatitis and pancreatitis. Carbamazepine may worsen seizures and cause cardiac rhythm disturbances. Ethosuximide may cause movement disorders such as dyskinesia and bradykinesia. Drugs should not be discontin-

ued abruptly because this can precipitate seizures.

Drug Interactions

- Sedative effects are enhanced by drugs that also have sedative properties. Barbiturates can decrease the effectiveness of corticosteroids and anticoagulants.
- St. John's wort should be avoided, and drug actions can be affected by ginkgo and ginseng.

Implications for Physical Therapists

- Epileptic patients, even with drug treatment, are vulnerable to intense lights and sound, which can precipitate a seizure. Keep patients in a quiet area without flickering lights and repetitive noise.
- Inform patients that they should take the medication exactly as prescribed because only this will assure maximal antiepileptic effects. Tell patients not to stop medication abruptly because this can precipitate seizures. Also, if blood tests were ordered, have patients adhere to such schedule because early detection of a problem can often prevent detection through such tests or reverse pathological changes.
- If patients are too sedated for therapy, discuss this with them and schedule appointments at times when they feel less sedated.
- Watch out for unexplained rashes, and notify or have patients contact their physician immediately, because some drugs can cause Stevens-Johnson syndrome. This necessitates immediate drug withdrawal.
- If patients should appear excessively sedated, have them contact a physician because a dosage change or other drug might be indicated.

Antidepressants

Common Drugs (selection of some of the most commonly used drugs)

Tricyclics
Amitriptyline (Elavil, Endep, other)
Amoxapine (Asendin)
Clomipramine (Anafranil)
Desipramine (Norpramin)
Doxepin (Sinequan)
Imipramine (Norfranil, Tofranil, other)
Nortriptyline (Aventyl, Pamelor)
Trimipramine (Surmontil)
Monoamine oxidase (MAO) inhibitors
Phenelzine (Nardil)
Tranylcypromine (Parnate)
Second generation
Bupropion (Wellbutrin)
Citalopram (Celexa)
Escitalopram (Lexapro)
Fluoxetine (Prozac)
Fluvoxamine (Luvox)
Mirtazapine (Remeron)
Paroxetine (Paxil)
Sertraline (Zoloft)
Trazodone (Desyrel)
Venlafaxine (Effexor)
Antimanic drug
Lithium

Indications

Antidepressants are indicated in:

- *Depression*, which can be roughly divided into unipolar and bipolar depression. Unipolar depression is characterized by dysphoria, lack of interest, fatigue, lack of energy, low self-esteem, irrational guilt, and suicidal ideation. Bipolar depression is characterized by swings between depression and mania. Mania is characterized by endless energy, increased activity, excessive euphoria, extreme irritability, racing thoughts, and fast talking, with little sleep needed, unrealistic beliefs in one's abilities and powers, poor judgment, and aggressive behavior. It is hypothesized that these disorders are caused mostly by a pathological supersensitivity of the pre- and postsynaptic receptors of the norepinephrine, serotonin, and dopamine systems. Drugs seem to increase synaptic neurotransmitter levels, down-regulate these receptors, normalize excessive receptor sensitivity, and improve mood. Receptor down-regulation might be the major effect because this takes time, which coincides with the delayed mood improvement that usually occurs after 4 to 6 weeks of therapy. The tricyclic drugs act by blocking the reuptake of all of the three neurotransmitters—albeit slightly differently. The MAO inhibitors inhibit the enzyme that decreases neurotransmitter destruction and increases intraneuronal levels and release. They affect both enzyme types (A&B), although inhibition of type A seems to be more beneficial. The second-generation drugs are also reuptake inhibitors but are somewhat more selective in their actions. These drugs include the selective serotonin reuptake inhibitors (SSRIs) such as fluoxetine, citalopram, escitalopram, fluoxamine, paroxetine, and sertraline, which mostly affect serotonin. Lithium is used mostly to prevent mood swings in bipolar depression, and its action is uncertain, but it might involve an action on neuronal excitability and the formation and action of certain second messengers.

- *Chronic pain* (neuropathic pain, fibromyalgia, chronic low back pain), which involves some of the above-mentioned neurotransmitters, particularly serotonin. However, the specific action of the drugs in this condition is unknown.

- Other conditions like *enuresis* (based on anticholinergic properties), *migraine, premenstrual disorder, attention deficit–hyperactivity disorder or ADHD, obsessive-compulsive disorders* (fluoxetine, sertraline), *anxiety disorders* (venlafaxine), and *smoking cessation* (bupropion). Mechanisms are often poorly understood.

Examples of Common Dosages
(general guidelines, many different dosage schedules)

Amitriptyline: 75–150 mg/day in divided doses PO (not to exceed 300 mg/day)

Amoxapine: 50–100 mg 2–3 times daily PO (not to exceed 300 mg/day)

Clomipramine: 25–250 mg in divided doses daily PO

Desipramine: 100–200 mg/day in divided doses up to 300 mg/day PO

Doxepin: 25–75 mg/day in divided doses up to 300 mg/day PO

Imipramine: 75–100 mg/day up to 300 mg/day in divided doses PO

Nortriptyline: 25 mg up to -150 mg/day in divided doses PO

Trimipramine: 50–200 mg/day in divided doses PO

Phenelzine: 45–60 mg/day in divided doses PO

Tranylcypromine: 10–30 mg 2 times daily PO

Bupropion: 100–150 mg 2–3 times daily PO

Citalopram: 20–40 mg/day once daily PO

Escitalopram: 10–20 mg/day once daily PO

Fluoxetine: 20 mg 1–2 times daily (not to exceed 80 mg/day) PO

Fluvoxamine: 50–100 mg 1–2 times daily (not to exceed 300 mg/day) PO

Mirtazapine: 15–45 mg once daily PO

Paroxetine: 20–60 mg once daily PO

Sertraline: 50–200 mg once daily PO

Trazodone: 150–600 mg in divided doses daily PO

Venlafaxine: 75–150 mg 2–3 times daily PO

Lithium: 300–600 mg 3 times daily PO

Administration

Most drugs are given PO.

Contraindications

Drugs should not be used or must be used with caution in patients with strong suicidal tendencies, seizure disorders, cardiac problems, and hepatic and renal diseases.

Common Adverse Reactions

Adverse reactions differ among the three groups, but patients are generally at higher risk of committing suicide at the beginning of therapy with all drugs. Also, long-term therapy will lead to different degrees of physical dependence, causing withdrawal syndrome (fatigue, headache, muscle pain) at abrupt drug therapy cessation. Tricyclics cause sedation, anticholinergic effects, orthostatic hypotension, cardiac dysrhythmias, and seizures, although there are differences among individual drugs. Occurrence of blood disorders (agranulocytosis) is rare but can be serious. MAO inhibitors show fewer of these effects, except a tendency for orthostatic hypotension. Second-generation drugs show seizure possibilities but fewer of the other adverse reactions, except for maprotiline, mirtazapine, nefazodone, and trazodone, which are similar to the tricyclics. A few of the latter drugs may cause malignant hyperthermia. Lithium has a very small margin of safety requiring periodic blood level tests to avoid serious toxicity. Some adverse reactions include confusion, lethargy, ataxia, increased deep tendon reflexes, and a fine tremor, and at higher doses, seizures and coma.

Drug Interactions

- Some drugs can interact with MAO inhibitors, resulting in seizures and hypertension, as well as with a large number of other drugs such as benzodiazepines and alcohol, resulting in enhanced sedation.
- Salt intake can affect lithium's effectiveness, and salt intake should not be changed during lithium therapy.
- MAO inhibitors can cause a severe hypertensive crisis with chest pain, headache, and nausea when taken with foods and drinks containing the chemical tyramine.
- Drugs can show increased toxicity with many herbs including St. John' wort, chamomile, valerian, and jimson weed. Increased toxicity of antidepressants occurs with methionine supplements.

Implications for Physical Therapists

- If patients complain about not feeling the beneficial effects of drug therapy in the first few weeks, advise them that it might take up to 6 weeks before they notice beneficial effects.
- If a patient should talk about "life is not worth living" in the beginning of therapy, notify a physician immediately as there is an increased risk of suicide during this time.
- If a patient receiving long-term therapy plans to discontinue the drug without advice of the physician, warn the patient and contact the physician because the possibility of a serious withdrawal reaction exists.
- If a patient taking lithium talks incessantly, becomes easily irritated, or becomes aggressive, notify a physician because this might require a change in dosage.
- Advise patients to change positions or get up slowly because some drugs can cause marked orthostatic hypotension.
- Advise patients taking lithium to strictly follow their physician's advice in taking the drug as prescribed and in having blood levels checked periodically. Should you notice tremors, lethargy, hyper-reflexia, and ataxia, notify the physician immediately because this may require dosage adjustments.
- Ask older patients if they have trouble voiding and have regular bowel movements, because some drugs with anticholinergic properties can cause urinary hesitancy and significant constipation. Advise these patients to increase water and bulk food intake to prevent constipation and its possible complications.

Antiemetics

Common Drugs (selection of some of the most commonly used drugs)

Serotonin 3 antagonists
  Dolasetron (Anzemet)
  Ondansetron (Zofran)
  Other
Histamine antagonists
  Dimenhydrinate (Dramamine, Gravol, other [OTC])
  Meclizine (Antivert, Antrizine, other [OTC])
  Other
Phenothiazines
  Chlorpromazine (Thorazine)
  Prochlorperazine (Compazine, other)
  Promethazine (Phenadoz)
  Other
Cholinergic antagonists
  Scopolamine
  Other
Miscellaneous drugs
  Metoclopramide (Reglan, other)
  Other

Indications

Antiemetics are indicated in:

* *Prevention and therapy of nausea and vomiting.* Serotonin antagonists block the stimulatory action of serotonin on type 3 receptors in the stomach and brain, reducing nausea and vomiting. Histamine antagonists block the action of histamine on H1 receptors in the periphery and, presumably with their cholinergic-blocking activity, inhibit central activity in the vestibular system as well as the chemoreceptor trigger zone and vomiting center. The phenothiazines seem to exert their action mostly via blockade of dopamine, histamine, and acetylcholine receptors. Metoclopramide seems to block dopamine receptors in the chemoreceptor trigger zone and increase gastric emptying time.
* *Motion sickness* (histamine antagonists, scopolamine) mostly one hour before exposure.

Examples of Common Dosages
(general guidelines, many different dosage schedules)

Dolasetron: 100 mg once PO, or 1.8 mg/kg once IV
Ondansetron: 8 mg to be repeated when needed PO, or 0.15 mg/kg to be repeated if needed IV
Dimenhydrinate: 50–100 mg every 4 hrs PO
Meclizine: 25–100 mg daily in divided doses PO
Chlorpromazine: 10–25 mg every 4–6 hrs PO, or 25–50 mg every 3 hrs IM
Prochlorperazine: 5–10 mg 3–4 times PO
Promethazine: 12.5–25 mg every 4–6 hrs PO, IM, IV, or rectally
Scopolamine: 1.5 mg transdermal (patch)
Metoclopramide: 1–2 mg/kg can be repeated IV

Administration

Depending on the drug, they can be given PO, IV, IM, or rectally. Scopolamine is used as a patch behind the ear.

Contraindications

Drugs are contraindicated (or should be used with caution) in older patients. (See *Antipsychotics* and *Anticholinergics*).

Common Adverse Reactions

Most drugs cause sedation and drowsiness. Serotonin antagonists can cause musculoskeletal pain, dysrhythmias, and, rarely, bronchospasm. Histamine antagonists cause confusion (mainly in geriatric individuals), dry mouth and eyes, and constipation. The phenothiazines can cause a number of adverse effects (see Antipsychotics). Scopolamine causes anticholinergic effects (see *Anticholinergics*). Metoclopramide can cause seizures and suicidal ideation.

Drug Interactions

Serotonin antagonists show few interactions. Histamine antagonists show enhanced anticholinergic activity with all drugs that also have these effects. Phenothiazines show a series of interactions (see *Antipsychotics*).

Implications for Physical Therapists

Observe patients for signs of dizziness and drowsiness, particularly older individuals, and be close by to prevent falls. In the case of phenothiazines, be aware of orthostatic hypotension.

Antifungals

Common Drugs (selection of some of the most commonly used drugs)

Amphotericin B (Fungizone, Abelcet, other)
Azole drugs
    Clotrimazole (Mycelex, Lotrim, other [OTC])
    Itraconazole (Sporanox)
    Miconazole (Moristat, other)
    Other
Miscellaneous drugs
    Griseofulvin (Grifulvin, other)
    Nystatin (Nilstat, Nystex, other)
    Tolnaftate (Tinactin, Aftate, other)
    Other

Indications

Antifungal drugs are indicated in:

- *Topical and systemic fungal infections affecting skin, vagina, nails, lungs, and other parts of the body.* Amphotericin B, which is specific for the fungal membrane, binds to ergosterol and forms with it a channel through which necessary nutrients escape, leading to the death of the fungus. Azole drugs inhibit the enzyme that synthesizes ergosterol. This reduces formation of a firm membrane and leads to the loss of nutrients and the death of the fungus. Nystatin acts in a similar way to amphotericin B; griseofulvin binds to fungal mitotic spindles during division and interferes with replication; and tolnaftate acts by an unknown mechanism.

- Drugs are fungus specific, and must often be taken for long periods of time and exactly as prescribed to be fully effective.

Drug resistance is not a major problem at this time.

- Some examples are systemic aspergillosis, candidiasis, cryptococcosis, and histoplasmosis, which are treated with amphotericin B as the primary drug, and sometimes with itraconazole as a secondary medication; tinea infections ("ring worm") with tolnaftate or clotrimazole; vulvovaginal candidiasis with clotrimazole; infections of scalp, skin and toes with griseofulvin; and oropharyngeal candidiasis with nystatin.

Examples of Common Dosages
(general guidelines, many different dosage schedules)

Amphotericin B: 0.25–0.5 mg/kg IV
Clotrimazole: Topical preparations
Itraconazole: 200–400 mg daily PO
Miconazole: Topical preparations
Griseofulvin: 500–1000 mg daily PO
Nystatin: Topical preparations and 500,000–1,000,000 units 3 times daily PO
Tolnaftate: Topical preparations

Administration

Amphotericin B is usually given by slow infusion, with test doses preceding the actual therapeutic amounts. The other drugs are mostly given topically or orally.

Contraindications

Drugs are contraindicated (or should be used with caution) in patients with renal and hepatic disorders.

Common Adverse Reactions

Amphotericin B is quite toxic and can cause seizures, renal toxicity, blood disorders, and allergic reactions. The other drugs, when given topically, show few adverse reactions. Oral administrations carry a higher risk with nausea, vomiting, and abdominal discomfort. Itraconazole can cause muscle pain and hepatotoxicity.

Drug Interactions

- Depending on the drug, the azole drugs can interfere with the biotransformation of other drugs and can increase each other's toxicity.
- Gossypol increases itraconazole's nephrotoxicity.

Implications for Physical Therapists

- Advise patients who use OTC antifungal preparations to contact a physician because successful therapy of fungal infections can be complex.
- Observe patients who take drugs that can be hepatotoxic for skin and eye color, and contact or have patients inform their physician if you notice yellowing of skin or eyes, which could be drug-induced liver toxicity.
- If you notice redness between the toes of a patient, contact or have the patient contact a physician as this could be a tinea infection (athlete's foot). If this is a school child or student, or a person using a locker room, you should also contact those facilities and have them disinfect the locker rooms.

Antihelminthics

Common Drugs (selection of some of the most commonly used drugs)

Albendazole (Albenza)
Mebendazole (Vermox)
Praziquantel (Biltricide)
Pyrantel (Antiminth, Ascarel, other)
Other

Indications

Antihelminthic drugs are indicated in:

- *Tape worm infections.* These are treated with praziquantal and albendazole, which paralyze the worms.
- *Fluke infections.* These are treated with praziquantal, which paralyzes the flukes.
- *Trichinosis and other infections.* These are treated with albendazole or mebendazole, which deprive the worms of glucose and other nutrients.

Examples of Common Dosages
(general guidelines, many different dosage schedules)

Albendazole: 400 mg 2 times daily PO
Mebendazole: 100 mg 1–2 times a day for 3 days PO
Praziquantel: 20 mg/kg 3 times a day PO
Pyrantel: 11 mg/kg once, or for 3 days PO

Administration

Depending on the drug, they are given mostly PO.

Contraindications

Drugs are contraindicated (or should be used with caution) in patients with hepatic diseases.

Common Adverse Reactions

In general, drugs may cause nausea, headache, abdominal discomfort, and diarrhea (in addition to the effects of a laxative, which is often prescribed to help expel intestinal worms). Albendazole and mebendazole can be hepatotoxic.

Drug Interactions

Few serious interactions are noticeable except with some drugs, including cimetidine (OTC), which increase the concentration of albendazole in tissue.

Implications for Physical Therapists

- If a patient with a worm infection is treated, wear gloves and wash hands thoroughly after therapy because eggs can spread easily. If he or she uses the toilet, have the toilet cleaned with disinfectant soap.
- If you notice a yellow skin color or yellowing of the conjunctiva, contact or have the patient contact a physician because some drugs can cause liver problems.

Antihistaminics

Drugs (selection of some of the most commonly used drugs)

Antihistamines
    Cetirizine (Zyrtec)
    Desloratadine (Clarinex)
    Dimenhydrinate (Dramine [OTC])
    Diphenhydramine (Allermed, Benadryl, other [OTC])
    Fexofenadine (Allegra)
    Loratadine (Alavert, Claritin, other [OTC])
    Other
Mast Cell Stabilizer
    Cromolyn (Nasalcrom, other)
    Nedocromil (Tilade)

Indications

Drugs are indicated in

- *Type I allergy*, which is characterized by hives, redness, and itching, and is caused by allergen-induced excessive histamine release and its vasodilating and nerve-irritating action (quick onset). Typical antihistaminics block action of histamine on its receptor or replace already bound histamine from receptor. Mast cell stabilizers stabilize membranes and prevent histamine release from these cells Massive histamine release precipitates an anaphylactic reaction (bronchoconstriction, severe hypotension), which responds to epinephrine, causing vasoconstriction (alpha-receptor stimulation) and bronchorelaxation (beta-receptor stimulation). Corticosteroids are also used and act through vasoconstriction (see *Corticosteroids*).
- Other uses such as *motion sickness and nausea* (dimenhydrinate, diphenhydramine) and *Parkinson disease.*

Examples of Common Dosages
(general guidelines, many different dosage schedules)

Cetirizine: 5–10 mg/day PO
Desloratadine: 5 mg/day PO
Dimenhydrinate: 50–100 mg every 4–6 hrs PO
Diphenhydramine: 25–50 mg every 4–6 hrs PO
Fexofenadine: 60–180 mg/day PO
Loratadine: 10 mg/day PO
Cromolyn: 1 spray into each nostril not to exceed 6 sprays
Nedocromil: 2 inhalations 2–4 times per day

Administration

Drugs are administered PO except for inhalations of mast cell stabilizers.

Contraindications

Antihistamines should not be used, or should be used with caution, in benign prostatic hyperplasia, where they may interfere with urination. Mast cell stabilizers have few contraindications.

Adverse reactions

All antihistamines cause some sedation and drowsiness as well as anticholinergic effects (see *Anticholinergics*) but mostly with diphenhydramine. Hepatitis may occur with desloratadine, blood disorders (hemolytic anemia) have been reported with diphenhydramine and fexofenadine and dysrhythmias with fexofenadine. Mast cell stabilizers show few adverse reactions except some throat irritation.

Drug Interactions

- Enhanced sedation and anticholinergic effects may occur with drugs that also have these effects. Alcohol enhances the sedative actions. Drugs used at higher doses can interfere with a number of other drugs also given at high doses.
- Sedative and anticholinergic effects are increased by hops, seneca, and corkwood

Implications for Physical Therapists

- Drugs can produce some sedation and confusion (mostly in geriatric patients) and can interfere with therapy. Schedule appointments at the end of drug actions.
- Advise individuals who take OTC antihistaminics that they can interfere with urination in cases of benign prostatic hyperplasia in older men and can cause contact lens intolerance because of dry eyes. Self-medication is recommended for short periods of time only.
- Advise patients that diphenhydramine is not recommended by physicians to be used as a hypnotic because it does not cause a restful sleep.

Antilipidemics

Common Drugs (selection of some of the most commonly used drugs)

HMG-CoA reductase inhibitors
    Atorvastatin (Lipitor)
    Fluvastatin (Lescol)
    Lovastatin (Altocor, Mevacor)
    Rosuvastatin (Crestor)
    Simvastatin (Zocor)
Bile acid sequestrants
    Cholestyramine (LoCholest, Prevalite, other)
    Colesevelam (Welchol)
    Colestipol (Colestid)
Miscellaneous drugs
    Ezetimibe (Zetia)
    Fenofibrate (Antara, Lofibra, other)
    Gemfibrozil (Lopid)
    Niacin (Niac, Niaspan, other (also available [OTC]))
    (Also available as nicotinic acid and nicotinamide)

Indications

Antilipidemics are indicated in:

- *Dyslipidemias* (caused by genetic basis, diet, diseases such as diabetes, drugs), which are characterized by increased levels of cholesterol and/or triglycerides in the blood. If levels are permanently elevated, pathological changes can occur in blood vessels. Initiated by a chronic inflammatory response in the vessel walls partly because of the action of white blood cells, low-density lipoproteins deposit excessive amounts cholesterol and triglycerides that are not adequately removed. This leads to hardening of the arteries (arteriosclerosis) and the formation of plaques (atherosclerosis), which can narrow and finally block blood vessels. The hardening of blood vessels increases blood pressure and impairs the supply of nutrients and oxygen to tissues, including the heart and brain. Parts of these plaques can break loose and block subsequent smaller vessels. Small blood clots formed elsewhere can become stuck and block such narrowed vessels. These can be the causes for myocardial infarctions (MIs) and strokes. Although high cholesterol and lipid levels increase the risk of such events, they are only soft indicators, because some individuals with low cholesterol levels can have strokes and MIs and others with high levels might not.

- Drugs used in hypercholesterolemia and/or elevated triglyceride levels will lower cholesterol and lipid levels, thus reducing the risk of atherosclerosis and the sequelae of cardiac and central problems.
- The HMG-CoA reductase inhibitors reduce endogenous synthesis of cholesterol. The HMG-CoA reductase inhibitors are the most effective drugs and can lower cholesterol levels by about 30%. The bile acid sequestrants bind to cholesterol in the gut and prevent its absorption. Ezetimibe reduces the absorption of cholesterol from the gut. Fenofibrate increases lipolysis by activating lipoprotein lipase, which decreases triglyceride levels and changes the size of the LDLs, leading to their rapid breakdown. Gemfibrozil, by an uncertain mechanism, decreases triglyceride levels and interferes with the synthesis of VLDLs and LDLs. Niacin, or vitamin B3, reduces the release of fatty acids from fat, decreases LDLs, and, perhaps most significantly, seems to increase HDLs.

Examples of Common Dosages
(general guidelines, many different dosage schedules)

Atorvastatin: 10–80 mg once daily PO (not to exceed 80 mg/day)

Fluvastatin: 20–80 mg once or divided PO

Lovastatin: 20–80 mg in single or divided doses PO

Rosuvastatin: 5–40 mg daily PO

Simvastatin: 5–40 mg daily PO (not to exceed 80 mg/day)

Cholestyramine: 4 g twice a day up to 24 g/day PO

Colesevelam: 3 625 mg tabs twice a day PO

Colestipol: 2–8 g twice a day PO

Ezetimibe: 10 mg/day PO

Fenofibrate: 40–160 mg/day PO

Gemfibrozil: 600 mg twice a day PO

Niacin: 100–500 mg/day in divided doses PO

Administration

These drugs can be given IV or PO. Some of these drugs can be prescribed in combination.

Contraindications

These drugs should not be used or must be used with caution in individuals with hepatic diseases.

Common Adverse Reactions

- Common adverse reactions include headache, abdominal cramps, dizziness, and heartburn.
- In addition, HMG-CoA reductase inhibitors can cause lens opacities (eye examinations are warranted), liver dysfunction (frequent liver function tests are indicated in the beginning of therapy), muscle pain with rhabdomyolysis (breakdown of skeletal muscle), hemolytic anemia, and photosensitivity reactions. Bile acid sequestrants can cause constipation; fecal impact; flatulence; decreased absorption of vitamins A, D, and K, with increased risk of bleeding; red blood cell formation; and hyperchloremic acidosis (rapid breathing, confusion). Ezetimibe causes few major adverse reactions. Fenofibrate can cause dysrhythmias. Gemfibrozil can cause leucopenia and anemia. Niacin causes flushing, orthostatic hypotension, and sometimes hepatotoxicity (jaundice, dark urine).

Drug Interactions

HMG-CoA reductase inhibitors in the presence of some antifungal drugs, erythromycin, and niacin show an increased risk of rhabdomyolysis. Grapefruit juice may increase toxicity and St. John's wort and bran may decrease therapeutic response. Bile acid sequestrants can interfere with the absorption of many drugs.

Implications for Physical Therapists

- Ask patients—particularly if blood pressure is elevated and body weight high—if cholesterol levels have been checked in the past. If not, strongly advise patients to see a physician because high cholesterol levels can be a "silent" (no symptoms) killer.
- Warn patients not to self-medicate with OTC niacin because the use of niacin should be monitored by a physician. Niacin can cause liver damage. Blood tests are necessary during therapy, and early detection of such a problem can prevent liver damage.
- If patients are using HMG-CoA reductase inhibitors and complain about muscle pain or mention a darkening of the urine, contact or have them notify a physician immediately because this could be a sign of rhabdomyolysis.
- Tell patients to see a physician at scheduled intervals, particularly in the beginning of therapy, because special laboratory tests have to be made to assure that no adverse reactions (e.g., liver) manifest themselves with use of drugs such as niacin and

HMG-CoA reductase inhibitors. Early detection can prevent permanent damage.

- Advise patients that in addition to drug therapy, a diet low in cholesterol and fats should be followed, combined with some daily exercise and keeping body weight at a normal level.

Antineoplastics

Common Drugs (selection of some of the most commonly used drugs)

Alkylating agents
   Carmustine (BCNU, Gliadel)
   Cyclophosphamide (Cytoxan, Neosar)
   Mechlorethamine (Mustargen, Nitrogen Mustard)
   Other
Platinum containing compounds
   Cisplatin (Platinol)
   Other
Antimetabolites
   Fluorouracil (Adrucil, Efudex, other)
   Mercaptopurine (Purinethol)
   Methotrexate (Amethopterin, Folex, other)
Antibiotics
   Bleomycin (Blenoxane)
   Dactinomycin (Cosmegen)
   Doxorubicin (Adriamycin)
   Other
Plant alkaloids
   Etoposide (Vepeside, Etopophos)
   Paclitaxel (Taxol, Onxol)
   Topotecan (Hycamtin)
   Vincristine (Oncovin, Vincasar)
   Other
Hormonal drugs
   Estradiol (Estrace, Gynodiol)
   Testosterone (Andro, Testaqua, other)
   Other

Tyrosine kinase inhibitors
   Erlotinib (Tarceva)
   Other
Biological response modifiers
   Interferons (Roferon, Pegintron, other)
   Rituximab (Rituxan)
   Other
Other drugs
   Hydroxyurea (Droxia, Hydrea)
   Other

Indications

Antineoplastics are indicated in:

- *All types of tumors and cancers.* Drugs interfere selectively with different steps in DNA synthesis, cell division, and growth. Alkylating agents bind covalently to two opposite bases and crosslink the two DNA strands together so that they cannot separate. Platinum-containing compounds also cross-link DNA strands. Antimetabolites are drugs that are structurally similar to some of the endogenous bases necessary for DNA synthesis. They are either incorporated into the DNA chain, where they produce a nonfunctioning base or DNA sequence, or they inhibit the enzymes that form the endogenous bases from precursors. Antibiotics act in different and often poorly understood ways and might be inserted into DNA strands, causing strand splitting; inhibiting DNA-related enzymes; forming highly toxic radicals; and/or disturbing the cell walls of cancer cells. Plant alkaloids are either antimitotic drugs that bind to and disrupt the function of the microtubules, which are necessary for cell division, or they are enzyme inhibitors that inhibit certain enzymes (e.g., topoisomerases), causing a break in the DNA strands. Hormonal drugs are used in cancers that are hormone stimulated (such as estrogen synthesis inhibitors in estrogen-sensitive breast cancer, or antiandrogens in androgen-promoted prostate cancer). Tyrosine kinase inhibitors affect a special tyrosine kinase enzyme that participates in the rapid cell division of neoplastic cells. Biological response modifiers are interleukins, interferons, and monoclonal antibodies (ending in -mab), which among other actions stimulate the body's immune system to fight such cells. The specific drug used depends on the type of neoplasm to be treated. Often, "cocktails" or mixtures of two to five drugs are prescribed to increase "total cell kill."

- Other uses such as *keratoses* (fluorouracil) and *ulcerative colitis and psoriatic arthritis* (mercaptopurine).

Examples of Common Dosages
(general guidelines, many different dosage schedules)

Carmustine: 150–200 mg/m^2 single dose every 6 weeks IV

Cyclophosphamide: 1–5 mg/kg/day or 40–50 mg/kg in divided doses over 2–5 days IV

Mechlorethamine: 0.4 mg/kg as single or divided doses over 2–4 days IV

Cisplatin: 20–100 mg/m^2 once or for several days every 3–4 weeks IV

Fluorouracil: 370–425 mg/m^2 daily for 5 days IV

Mercaptopurine: 2.5–5 mg/kg/day PO

Methotrexate: 15–30 mg/day for 5 days PO, IM, or 40 mg/m^2 IV

Bleomycin: 0.25–0.5 units/kg 1–2 times weekly SC, IV, IM, or 15 units 2 times weekly IV

Dactinomycin: 500 mcg/m^2/day for 5 days to be repeated IV

Doxorubicin: 60–75 mg/m^2 3 times a week IV

Etoposide: 50–100 mg/m^2 for 5 days to be repeated every 3–4 weeks IV

Paclitaxel: 175 mg/m^2 over 3 hrs every 3 weeks for 4 courses IV

Topotecan: 1.5 mg/m^2/day for 5 days IV

Vincristine: 10–30 mcg/kg, may be repeated weekly IV

Estradiol: 10 mg 3 times daily or 1–2 mg 3 times daily PO

Testosterone: 25–100 mg 2–3 times a week IM

Erlotinib: 150 mg daily PO

Interferons: Many different schedules depending on interferon

Rituximab: 375 mg/m^2 once weekly for 4–8 doses IV

Hydroxyurea: 80 mg/kg single dose every 3 days PO

Administration

Depending on the drug, they can be given PO, IV, intracavitary, intrapericardial, or by infusion. A drug schedule usually involves a combination of two to five drugs to be administered repeatedly, with intervals often depending on how well the patient tolerates this therapy.

Contraindications

Drugs are contraindicated (or should be used with caution) in patients with infections, anemia, or ulcers. Because neoplasms can be fatal, therapy usually overrides all possible contraindications.

Common Adverse Reactions

Many adverse reactions are shared by antineoplastic drugs and are caused by interference with DNA synthesis and multiplication of healthy but rapidly dividing cells. Hair formation is inhibited in the hair follicles, resulting in hair loss. Suppression of bone marrow leads to a paucity of erythrocytes, causing anemia; of platelets, causing bleeding episodes; and of leukocytes, causing a decrease in immune activity and an increased risk of infections. These adverse reactions can be counteracted (see Hemopoietic Drugs and Immunomodulators). Effects on the GI system cause nausea, vomiting, diarrhea, lesions, and ulcers. Antidiarrheal drugs and antiemetic drugs can provide relief (see Antiemetics). Fatigue is commonly encountered with these drugs. Fortunately many of these adverse reactions are reversed when drug therapy is stopped. Renal, cardiac, and hepatic toxicities can also occur. Different chemotherapeutic drugs will show their own toxicities, such as pulmonary fibrosis, seizures, and allergic reactions including anaphylaxis.

Drug Interactions

Depending on the drug, many interactions are possible, particularly with drugs that weaken the immune system, increase blood clotting time, and cause anemia. NSAIDs increase GI problems.

Implications for Physical Therapists

- Inquire about unusual bleeding episodes (bruising, gum bleeding) and touch patients gently, because their blood-clotting ability might be seriously impaired. If such hemorrhagic episodes are present, inform or have patients contact their physician.
- Do not treat patients if you have an infectious disease, because their immune systems are weakened. Also inform patients that they should avoid public, crowded places, because these can increase the risk of an infection.
- Assess patients' breathing abilities because drugs can affect the lungs. If impairment is noticed, inform or have patients contact or inform physician.
- Many cancers involve pain and the use of pain medication. Use of massages, heat, and transcutaneous electrical nerve stimulation can provide some relief and reduce the need for pain medications.
- The physical therapist can encourage patients by assuring

them that many cancers can now be cured or placed into long-lasting remission, and that most of the adverse reactions will disappear after cessation of therapy.

Antiprotozoals

Common Drugs (selection of some of the most commonly used drugs)

Chloroquine (Aralen)
Mefloquine (Lariam)
Metronidazole (Flagyl, Protostat)
Primaquine (Primaquine)
Pyrimethamine (Daraprim, Fansidar [with sulfadoxine])
Other

Indications

Antiprotozoal drugs are indicated in:

- *Malaria*, which is a mosquito-borne disease caused by the *Plasmodium* species of protozoa. These parasites enter the human blood stream via a female mosquito bite, and are also later taken up from the blood by the mosquito to be introduced into other humans. Different species cause different problems, ranging from mild to severe forms of the disease. They accumulate in the liver and red blood cells, where they feed on hemoglobin and multiply. Chloroquine and mefloquine bind to the DNA of the parasites and interfere with its transcription, as well as inhibit the parasitic enzyme heme polymerase, which inactivates free heme, which is toxic to the parasite. Some species have become resistant to the drug. Pyrimethamine is a folate antagonist with a higher affinity for the parasite than the host's folate metabolism. Primaquine acts through uncertain mechanisms, perhaps killing by impairing the DNA function of the exo-red blood cell forms of the parasite in the liver. Metronidazole is believed to be metabolized to a substance that binds to and inhibits parasitic DNA synthesis. Other drugs are available as well. Parasites are becoming more resistant to drug therapy.

- *Amoebiasis* is caused by an amoeba, resulting in mild to severe diarrhea. Trichomoniasis is a protozoal infection of the vagina (men usually remain asymptomatic). Metronidazole is used in both cases, and metronidazole also has antibacterial activity. The drug is believed to be metabolized to a substance that binds to and inhibits parasitic DNA synthesis. The drug is relatively nontoxic.

- *Acanthamoeba keratitis* (red, painful eyes bothered by light) is caused by acanthamoeba living in dirty water and in nonsterile solutions used for cleaning contact lenses. Therapy includes use of itraconazole, polymyxin and/or neomycin, or polymyxin B (see Antifungal Drugs) for prolonged periods, sometimes months.

- *Toxoplasma gondii* is a protozoal infection transmitted to humans via cat feces or contaminated meat. Drugs of choice are pyrimethamine—sulfadiazine, which interfere with protozoal folic acid metabolism.
- *Other protozoal infections* that are mostly present outside the United States.
- Other uses, such as in *rheumatoid arthritis* (chloroquine).

Examples of Common Dosages
(general guidelines, many different dosage schedules)

Chloroquine: 5 mg/kg/wk 1–2 wks before exposure and for 8 wks after leaving the endemic area PO

Mefloquine: 1250 mg once not to be repeated PO

Metronidazole: 250 mg 3 times daily for 7 days PO, or 2 g once PO

Primaquine: 15 mg daily PO

Pyrimethamine: 100 mg followed by 25 mg/day for 4–5 wks PO

Administration
Depending on the drug, they can be administered IM or PO.

Contraindications
Drugs are contraindicated (or should be used with caution) in blood disorders that are treated with antimalarial drugs.

Common Adverse Reactions
Most drugs are tolerated relatively well, and most adverse reactions are observed after high-dose and long-term therapy. Chloroquine can affect the retina and heart, and primaquine might cause hemolytic anemia in susceptible individuals. Metronidazole is associated with bone marrow depression and seizures. Pyrimethamine might cause seizures, agranulocytosis, and respiratory problems.

Drug Interactions
- Antimalarials show few interactions with other drugs.
- Folic acid supplements might decrease action of folate inhibitors. Acidophilus should not be taken simultaneously with metronidazole.

Implications for Physical Therapists
- Inquire about the color of the urine in patients on primaquine because this drug can cause hemolytic anemia. If color changes are noted, contact or have patients inform their physician.
- If a patient on chloroquine therapy mentions visual disturbances, contact or have patient inform a physician, because this drug can damage the retina.
- Advise contact lens wearers to use sterile solutions and be careful in cleaning contact lenses, because an acanthamoeba infection is very difficult to treat and carries certain health risks that can be easily prevented.

Antipsychotics

Common Drugs (selection of some of the most commonly used drugs)

Phenothiazines
    Chlorpromazine (Thorazine, other)
    Fluphenazine (Prolixin, Moditen)
    Perphenzine (Perphenzine, Trilafon)
    Prochlorperazine (Chlorpazine, Compazine, other)
    Thioridazine (Mellaril)
    Thiothixene (Navane [rarely used])
    Trifluoperazine (Stelazine, Suprazine, other)

Butyrophenone
    Haloperidol (Haldol)

Miscellaneous
    Aripiprazole (Abilify)
    Clozapine (Clozaril)
    Loxapine (Loxitane)
    Olanzapine (Zydis, Zyprexa)
    Paliperidone (Invega)
    Quetiapine (Seroquel)
    Risperidone (Risperdal)
    Ziprasidone (Geodon)

Indications

Antipsychotics are indicated in:

- *Schizophrenia*, which is characterized by delusions, hallucinations, thought disorders (positive symptoms), reduced emotions, reduced social contact, reduced speech, and reduced pleasure (negative symptoms). Studies have shown the brains of schizophrenic patients to show certain abnormalities such as enlarged cerebral ventricles, a decreased number of synaptic connections in the prefrontal cortex, and an increased or decreased functioning of dopamine D2 and D3 receptors, depending on the area. All drugs seem to affect a number of neurotransmitters, but they also seem to cause a blockade of dopaminergic receptors (mostly D2), which is thought to cause an up-regulation of critical receptor activities as the true action, explaining its delayed therapeutic action by about 4 weeks. Typical antipsychotics also affect other receptors that are more involved in adverse reactions such as the blockade of α receptors with a decrease in blood pressure; of cholinergic receptors with occurrence of dry mouth and blurred vision (see *Cholinergic Agonists* or *Anticholinergics*); and of dopamine receptors in the basal ganglia with movement disorders (see *CNS Dopaminergic Agonists*). They mostly alleviate positive symptoms. The atypical antipsychotic drugs do not block dopaminergic receptors as much, but they are more significant in inhibiting serotonergic receptors in a relatively unknown way. They alleviate some of both positive and negative symptoms. Clinically, about one third of patients improve markedly, one third improve somewhat, and one third do not respond.
- Other uses for individual drugs include *depression* (see

Antidepressants), *dementia* in older individuals (thioridazine), *nausea* (see *Antiemetics*), *Tourette's syndrome* and mania (see *Antidepressants*).

Examples of Common Dosages
(general guidelines, many different dosage schedules)

Chlorpromazine: 10–50 mg every 2 hr with a gradual increase up to 2 g/day PO

Fluphenazine: 2.5–10 mg in divided doses up to 40 mg/day PO

Perphenazine: 8–16 mg in divided doses up to 64 mg/day PO

Prochlorperazine: 5–10 mg 3–4 times a day up to 150 mg/day PO

Thioridazine: 25–100 mg 3 times a day up to 800 mg/day PO

Thiothixene: 2–5 mg 2–3 times a day up to 30 mg/day PO

Trifluoperazine: 2–5 mg 2 times daily up to about 40 mg/day PO

Haloperidol: 0.5–5 mg 2–3 times daily up to 100 mg/day PO

Aripiprazole: 10–15 mg/day up to 30 mg/day PO

Clozapine: 300–600 mg in divided doses PO

Loxapine: 10 mg 2–4 times daily up to 100 mg/day PO

Olanzapine: 5–10 mg/day up to 15 mg/day PO

Paliperidone: 6 mg/day PO

Quetiapine: 25 mg 2 times daily up to 300 mg/day PO

Risperidone: 1 mg 2 times a day up to about 3 mg PO

Ziprasidone: 20 mg 2 times daily up to 80 mg/day PO

Administration
These drugs can be given PO or IV, including depot preparations, because psychotic patients often refuse to take the medication as prescribed.

Contraindications
Drugs should not be used or must be used with caution in patients with hepatic disorders, hyper- or hypotension, and cerebral arteriosclerosis.

Common Adverse Reactions
Common adverse reactions for most drugs include sedation and dizziness. Typical antipsychotics can cause pseudoparkinsonism, dystonia, akathisia, irreversible tardive dyskinesia, seizures, malignant hyperthermia, orthostatic hypotension, tachycardia, cardiac arrest, jaundice/hepatitis, constipation, urinary hesitancy, laryngospasm, respiratory depression, and, rarely, agranulocytosis. Some drugs interfere with body temperature regulation. Haloperidol has similar adverse reactions and seems to be less anticholinergic, but more dopaminergic. Atypical antipsychotics have similar adverse reactions but show fewer respiratory effects and a decreased risk of developing tardive dyskinesia.

Drug Interactions
- These drugs interact with a large number of drugs, particularly drugs with sedative, anticholinergic, and antihypertensive actions.

- Henbane leaves, nutmeg, and kava increase the drugs' toxicities.

Implications for Physical Therapists

- Patients might often not be cooperative or be fearful of novel environments and procedures, particularly if their paranoia is only partially controlled by drugs.
- Check patients for movement problems such as pseudoparkinsonism, dyskinesia, dystonia, akathisia, and tardive dyskinesia. If detected, inform physician directly because patients might not do so.
- Watch out for orthostatic hypotension with some of the drugs and have patients change positions slowly or avoid standing for long periods of time. Watch patients leaving a warm thera-

peutic pool because fainting is a possibility.
- Patients who are on medications with strong anticholinergic actions will show an increase in heart rate. Also advise chewing gum if a dry mouth becomes a disturbing problem.
- Ask older patients on drugs with strong anticholinergic actions if they experience constipation or urinary hesitance (mostly men). If yes, inform their physician to avoid complications of constipation or possible urinary retention.
- Check older patients who have received olanzapine IM for respiratory problems and notify a physician immediately if such problems are detected, to avoid the occurrence of pneumonia.

Antivirals

Common Drugs (selection of some of the most commonly used drugs)
DNA inhibitors
    Acyclovir (Zovirax)
    Famciclovir (Famvir)
    Foscarnet (Foscavir)
    Ganciclovir (Cytovene, Vitrasert)
    Valacyclovir (Valtrex)
    Other
Neuraminidase inhibitors
    Oseltamivir (Tamiflu)
    Other
Reverse transcriptase inhibitors
    Stavudine (Zerit)
    Tenofovir (Viread)
    Zidovudine (Retrovir)
    Other

Protease inhibitors
    Lopinavir (Kaletra [with ritonavir])
    Ritonavir (Norvir)
    Other
Miscellaneous action
    Amantadine (Symadine, Symmetrel)
    Enfuvirtide (Fuzeon)
    Interferons
Other

Indications

Antiviral drugs are indicated in:
- *Viral infections*. Viruses consist of single or double strands of DNA or RNA enclosed by a protein coat (capsid). They need the metabo-

lism of a specific host cell to multiply. The life cycle of a virus generally involves attachment to a host cell, penetration, shedding the protein coat, incorporation of viral DNA into the host cell DNA, formation of individual virus parts, cutting synthesized long proteins to virus size–needed protein (proteases), assembly of new viruses, and leaving the cell. Influenza viruses also need the enzyme neuraminidase to complete their biosynthesis and release. DNA inhibitors are first monophosphorylated (some by viral enzymes) and then di- and triphosphorylated by host-cell enzymes; the triphosphorylated compound is the active antiviral compound and competes with endogenous bases for DNA polymerase. It is partly incorporated as a "faulty" base, terminating viral DNA chain synthesis. Foscarnet works in a similar fashion but does not have to be phosphorylated. Neuraminidase inhibitors interfere with the completion of the synthesis and release of influenza viruses. Reverse transcriptase inhibitors affect RNA viruses; RNA is first transcribed into DNA by the enzyme reverse transcriptase, whose action is inhibited by these drugs, resulting in impairment of DNA synthesis and viral multiplication. Protease inhibitors prevent the cleavage of the long protein molecules into the smaller protein molecules necessary for viral assembly. Some drugs act by interfering with attachment/penetration and uncoating (amantadine, enfuvirtude), whereas others (interferons) protect neighboring cells from being infected. Vaccines can prevent many viral infections today.

- Drugs can be given prophylactically and therapeutically. Unfortunately, viruses become more and more resistant to these drugs by losing some of their special enzymes or by altering their DNA expression.

- Viral infections include: herpes infections; both initial and recurrent infections are treated with drugs such as acyclovir or valacyclovir. Herpes zoster infections are treated with famciclovir or valacyclovir. Influenza A and B infections are treated with oseltamivir (A and B) or amantadine (A). Cytomegalovirus infections are treated with ganciclovir. Chronic hepatitis can be treated with interferon α 2b or peginterferon α 2a. AIDS is treated mostly with reverse transcriptase inhibitors, protease inhibitors, and enfuvirtide.

- Drugs, mostly in combination, have to be given for long periods of time. During pregnancy they can prevent vertical transmission of the virus (from mother to fetus).

Examples of Common Dosages
(general guidelines, many different dosage schedules)

Acyclovir: 200–800 mg every 4 hrs PO

Famciclovir: 500 mg every 8 hrs PO

Foscarnet: 60 mg/kg given over 1 hr every 8 hrs for 2–3 wks IV

Ganciclovir: 1000 mg 3 times daily PO, or 5 mg/kg/dose given over 1 hr for 2–3 weeks IV

Valacyclovir: 1000 mg 3 times daily PO

Oseltamivir: 75 mg 2 times daily PO

Stavudine: 40 mg every 12 hrs PO

Tenofovir: 300 mg once daily PO

Zidovudine: 600 mg/day in divided doses, or 1–2 mg/kg every 4 hrs IV

Lopinavir: 400/100 mg 2 times daily, or 800/200 mg once daily PO

Ritonavir: 300 mg 2 times daily, followed by increased doses up to 600 mg 2 times daily PO

Amantadine: 200 mg/day, or 100 mg 2 times daily PO

Enfuvirtude: 90 mg 2 times daily SC

Interferons: Different schedules

Administration

Depending on the drug, they can be given PO, IV, SC, or topically (on blisters and eyes). Some must be injected into the eye.

Contraindications

Drugs are contraindicated (or should be used with caution) in patients with blood, renal, and hepatic disorders.

Common Adverse Reactions

Generally, most drugs can affect the kidneys, liver, and blood. Drugs taken at high doses might precipitate in the kidneys to form stones, which can be prevented by consuming large quantities of water. Neuralgia and myopathies may be encountered. Except for the reactions mentioned previously, DNA inhibitors are generally well-tolerated except foscarnet, which can cause cardiac arrest, acute renal failure, pulmonary embolism, and bronchospasm. Neuraminidase inhibitors such as oseltamivir may cause Stevens-Johnson syndrome. Reverse transcriptase inhibitors can cause blood dyscrasias and hepatotoxicity. Protease inhibitors may shift fat from other body places to the abdomen and cause insulin resistance, as well as increase cardiovascular risks. Amantadine has been associated with mood changes, loss of concentration in elderly individuals, and orthostatic hypotension; and enfuvirtide can cause neuropathy. Interferons have been associated with neuropsychiatric disorders, pancreatitis, dyscrasias, and autoimmune disorders.

Drug Interactions

- DNA inhibitors show few serious interactions. Drugs taken at high doses will interact with other drugs because of interference with renal excretion or metabolism. Some antiviral drugs interact with each other and when used simultaneously, administration must be spaced. Lopinavir and ritonavir interact with sildenafil and related drugs, and cause severe hypotension. Ritonavir interacts with a large number of drugs including St. John's wort, which decreases ritonavir's efficacy.

- Use of alcohol will increase toxicity of most drugs.

Implications for Physical Therapists

- If a skin rash is noticed, contact or have patients inform a physician, because some drugs can cause Stevens-Johnson syndrome.
- If you notice a yellow skin color or yellowing of conjunctiva, contact or have patients contact a physician as some drugs can be hepatotoxic.
- Emphasize that mothers should follow their physician's instructions and not breast-feed, because some drugs can pass through the milk into the child.

- Do not exercise patients who use lopinavir or ritonavir, and sildenafil and related drugs, because this might result in extreme hypotension and syncope.
- If patients have been instructed to drink large amounts of fluids, have them periodically drink water, particularly when they are sweating, to prevent formation of kidney stones.
- Emphasize to patients that open herpes blisters will transmit the virus by contact and advise abstinence from or use of condoms during intercourse.

Anxiolytics

Common Drugs (selection of some of the most commonly used drugs)

Benzodiazepines
  Alprazolam (Xanax)
  Chlordiazepoxide (Librium, other)
  Clonazepam (Klonopin)
  Clorazepate (Tranxene)
  Diazepam (Valium, other)
  Lorazepam (Ativan)
  Oxazepam (Serax)
Azapirone
  Buspirone (BuSpar)
Antidepressants (see Antidepressants)
  Doxepin
  Hydroxyzine
  Paroxetine
  Venlafaxine

Indications

Anxiolytics are mainly indicated in:

- *Anxiety disorders,* characterized by an excessive, irrational dread of every situation, can be disabling and significantly interfere with daily activities and functioning of the individual. There are five types: generalized anxiety disorder (chronic, exaggerated worry, tension, insomnia, irritability with no apparent cause), obsessive-compulsive disorder (urgent need to engage in certain rituals like being obsessed with germs or dirt and washing hands over and over again), panic disorder (pounding heart, chest pains, lightheadedness or dizziness, nausea, shortness of breath, fear of dying, sweating, feelings of unreality), post-traumatic stress disorder (persistent frightening thoughts and memories of past ordeals) and phobias (irrational fears of things, animals, or people).

- Benzodiazepines increase GABA action, increase hyperpolarization in adjacent nerve cells, reduce their neuronal firing, and dampen excessive neural activity, leading to a relatively quick reduction of anxiety. Buspirone also dampens excessive neuronal activity but through agonistic actions on the serotonin receptors, resulting in a delayed (2 to 4 weeks) antianxiety effect. Antidepressant drugs (see Antidepressants) affect depression, which is often associated with anxiety through actions on the norepinephrine and serotonergic system.
- Other conditions such as *premenstrual syndrome, depression, alcohol withdrawal, muscle relaxation, restless leg syndrome, seizure disorders*, and certain medical, diagnostic, and surgical procedures.

Examples of Common Dosages
(general guidelines, many different dosage schedules)

Alprazolam: 0.25–0.5 mg 3 times a day up to 4 mg/day PO
Chlordiazepoxide: 5–10 mg 3–4 times daily PO
Clonazepam: 1.5 mg/day in 3 divided dose PO (not to exceed 20 mg/day)
Diazepam: 2–10 mg 2–4 times daily PO
Lorazepam: 2–6 mg in divided doses up to 10 mg/day PO
Oxazepam: 10–30 mg 3–4 times daily up to 120 mg/day PO

Buspirone: 5 mg 3 times daily up to 60 mg/day PO

Administration
These drugs are given mostly PO but can also be injected IM or IV.

Contraindications
These drugs should not be used or must be used with caution in patients with a history of drug abuse and respiratory problems.

Common Adverse Reactions
Benzodiazepines will cause some sedation and psychomotor impairment. Less frequent are ECG changes, tachycardia, and agranulocytosis. Depending on the drug, they will all cause some physical dependence after long-term therapy and withdrawal symptoms (excitation, rebound anxiety, insomnia) might occur after abrupt cessation of therapy. Alprazolam must be withdrawn very slowly because convulsions might occur otherwise. Buspirone is almost devoid of adverse reactions except some dizziness and restlessness. Adverse reactions of the antidepressants are described in Antidepressants.

Drug Interactions
- Sedation caused by anxiolytics with sedative properties is increased by drugs that also have sedative actions.
- Sedative effects are increased by a number of herbs, including chamomile, mistletoe, and valerian. St. John's wort seems to reduce anxiolytic effectiveness.

Implications for Physical Therapists

- Physical therapists can be helpful in promoting nonpharmacological interventions such as relaxation techniques, excercises, or massages to reduce the use of anxiolytics.
- Patients on higher doses of benzodiazepines might have to be scheduled at times when the sedative and psychomotor impairments are less noticeable and will interfere less with therapy.
- Always watch older patients on benzodiazepine therapy for motor incoordination, sedation, and impaired gait, to avoid falls that can result in serious fractures.
- Advise patients at the start of buspirone therapy to be patient, as it can take about a month before anxiolytic effects become apparent.

β Agonists

Common Drugs (selection of some of the most commonly used drugs)

Beta 1 Agonists
   Dobutamine
Beta 2 Agonists (relatively selective)
   Albuterol (Salbutamol, Ventolin, Volmax, other)
   Formoterol (Foradil, Perforomist)
   Metaproterenol (Alupent)
   Pirbuterol (Maxair)
   Salmeterol (Serevent)
   Terbutaline (Brethine)
Beta 1 and 2 Agonists
   Isoproterenol
Mixed acting alpha and beta Agonist (see Alpha Agonists)

Indications

Beta agonists are indicated in:
- *Asthma*, in which bronchoconstriction (caused by allergy, exercise, cold air, or other conditions) decreases air flow and makes breathing difficult (wheezing). Selective beta 2 receptor agonists stimulate beta 2 receptors on bronchi, cause bronchi to dilate, and allow air to flow through bronchi more easily.
- *Chronic obstructive pulmonary disease* (COPD) and emphysema, in which air flow is impaired because of lung damage (as from smoking). Selective beta 2 receptor agonists stimulate beta 2 receptors on bronchi, cause bronchi to dilate, and allow air to flow through bronchi more easily.
- Other conditions such as *prevention of premature ventricular contractions* (ritodrine, terbutaline), *congestive heart failure* (dobutamine IV), or *severe hypotension* (dopamine IV).

Examples of Common Dosages (general guidelines, many different dosage schedules)

Albuterol: 2–4 mg 2–4 daily PO (not to exceed 32 mg/day), or 4–8 mg twice daily for extended release preparations, or 2–4 inhalations every 4–6 hr or 15 min before exercise

Formoterol: 1 cap (12 mcg) every 12 hr by inhalation

Metaproterenol: 20 mg 3–4 times daily PO

Metaproterenol: 1–2 inhalations every 4–6 hr (not to exceed 12 inhalations)

Salmeterol: 1 inhalation (50 mcg)

Terbutaline: 2.5–5 mg every 6–8 hr PO (not to exceed 15 mg/day)

Administration

These drugs can be given IV, PO, or by inhalation. Administration schedules vary among drugs because of differences in duration of action. Beta agonists are often combined with steroids (see Corticosteroids).

Contraindications

These drugs must be used with caution in cardiovascular disease, diabetes mellitus, and seizure disorders.

Common Adverse Reactions

Common adverse reactions include nervousness, restlessness, insomnia, tremor, chest pain, palpitations, increased blood pressure, and increased blood sugar levels. Excessive use of inhalers can lead to tolerance or paradoxical bronchospasm.

Drug Interactions

- They should not be used with MAO inhibitors.
- Caffeine in coffee or tea, figwort, and motherwort may enhance CNS effects.

Implications for Physical Therapists

- Be aware that exercise and cold air can aggravate asthma and bronchoconstriction. Have patients use inhaler 15 to 30 minutes before exercise depending on the drug, and avoid cold or drafty places.
- After inhalation or oral use, heart rate and blood pressure may increase. Patients with angina should be exercised slowly because beta agonists can increase risk of angina.
- If patients use inhalers too often, have patients notify their physician, because excessive use can cause tolerance or paradoxical bronchoconstriction.
- If patients show a fine tremor, notify or have patient contact the physician. The dose might have to be adjusted, or a different drug might have to be prescribed.

β Antagonists or Blockers

Common Drugs (selection of some of the most commonly used drugs)

Acebutolol (Sectral)
Atenolol (Tenormin)
Bisoprolol (Zebeta, Monocor)
Carteolol (Cartrol)

Carvedilol (Coreg)
Labetalol (Normodyne, Trandate)
Metoprolol (LopressorSR, Toprol-XL)
Nadolol (Corgard)
Penbutolol (Levatol)

Pindolol (Visken)
Propranolol (Inderal, InnoPranXL)
Sotalol (Betapace)

Indications

Beta antagonists or blockers are indicated in:

- *Angina*, where insufficient blood flow (e.g., atherosclerosis) does not supply enough oxygen to cardiac muscle, so that under emotional or physical stress heart rate and contractility increase. Cardiac needs now exceed the existing oxygen supply and cause anginal pain. Beta antagonists decrease heart rate and contractility, reducing the oxygen need and reducing or eliminating pain.

- *Hypertension* when blood pressure is increased above normal limits, leading to infarctions and strokes. Beta blockers lower blood pressure by reducing cardiac output (heart rate and contractility), blocking renin release, which reduces the formation of the vasoconstrictor angiotension and reducing via a central action sympathetic tone to blood vessels and heart.

- *Arrhythmias*, which are caused by abnormal electrical activity. Beta antagonists reduce overly excited cardiac activity and normalize heart rhythm (certain drugs only).

- *Tremors, migraine, anxiety, drug induced akathisia, aggressive behavior*, and other conditions where the mechanism of action is uncertain, but beta antagonists seem to be helpful.

- *Open-angle glaucoma*, in which intraocular pressure is elevated and may damage the retina, leading eventually to tunnel vision and blindness. Certain beta blockers (timolol, betaxolol, levobunalol) administered topically block the inflow of fluid into the eye and lower intraocular pressure.

Examples of Common Dosages

(general guidelines, many different dosage schedules)

Acebutolol: 400–800 mg/day once or twice (up to 1200 mg/day) PO

Atenolol: 25–100 mg once daily (up to 200 mg/day) PO

Bisoprolol: 5 mg once daily (up to 20 mg/day) PO

Carteolol: 2.5–10 mg once daily PO

Carvedilol: 3.125–6.25 mg twice daily (up to 50 mg daily) PO

Labetalol: 100–400 mg twice daily (up to 2.4 g daily) PO

Metoprolol: 25–100 mg/day as a single or divided dose (up to 450 mg/day) PO

Nadolol: 40–80 mg once daily (up to 320 mg/day) PO

Penbutolol: 20 mg once daily PO

Pindolol: 5 mg twice daily (up to 45–60 mg/day) PO

Propranolol: 40–320 mg/day single or divided daily PO

Sotalol: 80 mg twice daily (up to 320 mg) PO

Administration

These drugs can be given PO, IV, and, in some cases, topically into the eye. Long-term therapy must be stopped slowly or drug must be tapered to avoid withdrawal syndrome (cardiac problems).

Contraindications

These drugs must be used with caution in bradycardia, renal impairment, pulmonary disease (e.g., asthma), and diabetes mellitus.

Common Adverse Reactions

- Common adverse reactions include weakness, drowsiness, bradycardia, pulmonary edema, hypotension, impotence, and masking of hypoglycemic (in insulin-using patients by masking of tachycardia) and thyrotoxic episodes (e.g., masking of tachycardia).
- Topical administration causes fewer and milder systemic adverse reactions.

Drug Interactions

- May alter the effectiveness of insulin or hypoglycemics, antagonize use of beta agonists, and should not be used with MAO inhibitors.

Implications for Physical Therapists

- When exercising a patient, be aware that heart rate will be affected (reduced) by beta blockers.
- Advise patients to consult a physician if breathing difficulties are experienced during exercise, because drugs can cause bronchoconstriction and pulmonary edema.
- Have older patients get up slowly because drugs (mostly labetalol) can cause orthostatic hypotension, particularly at the beginning of therapy.
- Use exercise with caution in patients using insulin and beta blockers, because the beta blocker might mask the onset of a hypoglycemic episode.
- Patients taking beta blockers are sensitive to a cold environment and may experience cold extremities.
- Warn patients to not suddenly discontinue long-term beta-blocker use, because abrupt cessation can precipitate a serious withdrawal syndrome (including life-threatening arrhythmias).

Calcium Channel Blockers

Common Drugs (selection of some of the most commonly used drugs)

Amlodipine (Norvasc)

Diltiazem (Cardizem, Cartia XT, DilacorXR, other)

Felodipine (Plendil)

Isradipine (DynaCirc, DynaCirc CR)

Nicardipine (Cardene, Cardene SR)

Nifedipine (Adalat, Adalat CC, Procardia, Procardia XL)

Nisoldipine (Sular)

Verapamil (Apo-Verap, Calan, Isoptin, other)

Indications

Calcium channel blockers are indicated in:

- *Hypertension* or increased blood pressure, with increased risk of cardiac infarctions and strokes. Drugs block calcium fluxes in cardiac tissue and blood vessel walls, and reduce cardiac contractibility and relax blood vessels. This decreases cardiac output and peripheral resistance, and lowers blood pressure.

- *Angina pectoris*, when the oxygen demand of the compromised heart exceeds the oxygen supply from damaged coronary blood vessels. Drugs reduce contractibility, which reduces cardiac oxygen requirements; dilate coronary arteries to supply more blood and oxygen to the heart; and relax peripheral blood vessels, which decrease peripheral resistance, making it easier for the heart to eject the blood into the periphery (a special form is Prinzmetal angina, which is a spastic blood vessel constrictive form of angina).

- *Certain arrhythmias* such as supraventricular tachycardia, or atrial flutter and fibrillations. In these cases, electrical activity is conducted too fast or irregularly over the heart so that the cardiac muscle cannot contract completely and efficiently. Drugs reduce excitation-contraction coupling by slowing calcium movements, normalizing conduction, slowing the heart, and achieving more efficient contractions.

- *Congestive heart failure* (CHF), when the heart cannot pump enough blood to other organs of the body. This results in an enlarged heart, with the patient becoming quickly fatigued and short of breath (pulmonary edema) during even the slightest exertion. Drugs cause vasodilatation, which helps the heart to eject blood more easily and efficiently.

- *Migraine* with uncertain mechanism, and to prevent neurological damage because of cerebral blood vessel spasms (nimodipine).

Examples of Common Dosages
(general guidelines, many different dosage schedules)

Amlodipine: 5–10 mg once daily PO

Diltiazem: 30–120 mg 3–4 times daily PO, or 60–120 mg 2 times daily as S-capsules PO

Felodipine: 5–10 mg once a day PO

Isradipine: 2.5–10 mg twice daily PO, or 5–20 mg once daily as CR tablets PO

Nicardipine: 20–40 mg 3 times daily PO, or 30–60 mg 2 times daily with sustained release form PO

Nifedipine: 10–30 mg 3 times daily PO (not to exceed 180 mg/day), or 30–120 mg once daily with sustained release form PO

Nisoldipine: 20–60 mg once a day PO

Verapamil: 80–120 mg 3 times daily PO, or 120–240 mg once a day with extended release preparations PO

Administration

These drugs are given IV or PO. Dose must be adjusted in frail, geriatric patients and those with hepatic impairment.

Contraindications

These drugs are contraindicated (or to be used cautiously) in certain arrhythmias, hypotension, and congestive heart failure.

Common Adverse Reactions

These drugs can cause headache, certain arrhythmias, dizziness, peripheral edema, congestive heart failure, cough, joint stiffness, muscle cramps, and gingival hyperplasia (diltiazem). Rarely, they can cause Stevens-Johnson-syndrome.

Drug Interactions

- Hypotensive episodes may occur with nitrates, antihypertensives, and alcohol. Toxicity may be increased with use of H2 blockers.
- Grapefruit juice may reduce metabolism of some drugs and increase their blood serum levels, leading to overdose signs and symptoms. High-fat meals can increase blood levels of nisoldipine.

Implications for Physical Therapists

- Have patients change position and get up slowly, particularly in the beginning of therapy, because orthostatic hypotension may occur.
- Be careful when using a heated therapeutic pool, because warm water can aggravate the vasodilatory effects of peripheral vascular dilators and lead to a marked decrease in blood pressure.
- Observe patients for signs of congestive heart failure (peripheral edema, rales/crackles, dyspnea, weight gain, jugular venous extension), and if present, notify physician.
- Joint stiffness and muscle cramps are can be adverse reactions; notify the physician should these occur.
- If you notice peripheral edema, significant bradycardia or irregular heart beats, or swelling of gums, notify a physician.
- If patients feel feverish and exhibit an unexplained skin rash, ask them to immediately notify a physician, because this could be the onset of Stevens-Johnson syndrome and drugs should be stopped as soon as possible.

Cholinergic Agonists

Common Drugs (selection of some of the most commonly used drugs)

Cholinergic drugs
    Bethanechol (Duvoid, Urabeth, Urecholine)
    Pilocarpine (Akarpine, Pilocar, other)
    Neostigmine (Prostigmin)
    Pyridostigmine (Mestinon, Regonol)
    Other
Anti-Alzheimer drugs
    Donepezil (Aricept)
    Galantamine (Razadyne)

Rivastigmine (Exelon)
Tacrine (Cognex)
Memantine (Namenda)
Other

Indications

Cholinergic agonists are indicated in:

- *Postoperative gastrointestinal and urinary atony* (bethanechol). Drugs activate stimulatory muscarinic receptors and initiate intestinal or bladder activity.

- *Myasthenia gravis*, in which the number of cholinergic Nm receptors on skeletal muscles is decreased because of an autoimmune problem. Patients will show rapid fatigability and muscle weakness. Indirect-acting cholinergic agonists (neostigmine, pyridostigmine), through inhibiting the enzyme acetylcholinesterase and reducing acetylcholine destruction, can increase synaptic acetylcholine levels, which can now activate the remaining receptors and restore muscle activity.

- Dementia brought on by Alzheimer's disease, where it is believed that this condition is caused by a loss of nicotinic receptors (plus other abnormalities such as overstimulation of glutaminergic receptors). Again, indirect-acting cholinergic agonists can increase central synaptic acetylcholine levels, stimulate remaining nicotinic receptors, and slightly improve memory, but they will not alter the course of the disease. In addition, action of excessive glutamate is blocked by memantine, preventing damaging effects.

- *Reversal of effects of nondepolarizing neuromuscular blockers* by increasing synaptic acetylcholine levels, which compete with the blocker.

- *Glaucoma* (open-angle), where a defect in the trabecular outflow increases intraocular pressure, leading eventually to retinal damage, tunnel vision, and blindness. Cholinergic drugs (e.g., pilocarpine, isoflurophate) applied topically increase outflow and lower the damaging effects of an increased intraocular pressure.

Examples of Common Dosages
(general guidelines, many different dosage schedules)

Bethanechol: 25–50 mg three times daily PO

Donepezil: 5–10 mg once daily (not to exceed 5 mg in frail, geriatric women) PO

Galantamine: 4–12 mg twice daily PO (up to 24 mg)

Memantine: 5–10 mg 2 times daily PO

Neostigmine: 15 mg q 3–4 hr initially, which can be increased to 375 mg/day PO

Pyridostigmine: 30–60 mg q 3–4 hr, which can be increased to 600 mg/day PO or 180–540 mg 1–2 times daily for extended release preparations PO

Rivastigmine: 1.5 mg twice daily to be increased to 6 mg twice daily PO

Tacrine: 10 mg 4 times daily, which can be increased to 160 mg/day PO

Administration

These drugs are given PO, IM, and IV (or topically in the case of glaucoma). After topical administration, observed systemic adverse reactions are milder.

Contraindications

Contraindications include asthma, ulcer, cardiovascular disease, and epilepsy.

Common Adverse Reactions

Adverse reactions include bronchoconstriction with decreased airflow, headache, abdominal cramps, diarrhea (can cause dehydration), salivation, tearing, sweating, and bradycardia with heart block. Memantine might cause some drowsiness.

Drug Interactions

These drugs can antagonize the actions of anticholinergic drugs and may increase GI bleeding caused by NSAIDs. Jimson weed and Scopolia reduce their effectiveness.

Implications for Physical Therapists

- Drugs can reduce heart rate. The heart rate should be measured periodically, particularly during and after exercise.
- Drugs can cause dizziness, and patients, particularly older patients, must be observed when getting up, standing, or walking.
- If a patient is doing well on medication for myasthenia gravis but suddenly shows a reoccurrence of symptoms such as muscle weakness with some tremors, ask about their dosage. Taking too little or too much of the drugs (the latter is referred to as "myasthenic syndrome") can cause symptoms resembling the original condition, and the original dosage should be used again or the physician should be contacted.

CNS Dopaminergic Agonists

Common Drugs (selection of some of the most commonly used drugs)

Amantadine (Symmetrel)
Carbidopa-levodopa (Parcopa, Sinemet, other)
Entacapone (Comtan)
Pergolide (Permax)
Pramipexole (Mirapex)
Ropinirole (Requip)
Selegiline (Carbex, Eldepryl, other)
Tolcapone (Tasmar)
Other

Indications

CNS dopaminergic agonists are indicated in:

- *Parkinson disease*, which is a movement disorder characterized by a mask-like face, shuffling gait, and pill-rolling tremor. The cause is believed to be—among other problems—an overactivity of cholinergic and underactivity of dopaminergic activity in the basal ganglia of the brain. These drugs stimulate dopaminergic receptors directly (pergolide, pramipexole, ropinirole), increase the synthesis of dopamine (carbidopa), increase the release of dopamine (amantadine), or prevent the destruction of dopamine (selegiline, entacapone, tolcapone), which also leads to increased synaptic dopamine levels. This increase in dopaminergic activity restores the balance between the two neurotransmitter systems. One of these drugs (amantadine) is also an antiviral drug used for influenza A infections. Drugs that reduce cholinergic activity and restore imbalance as well are discussed under *Anticholinergics*.

Examples of Common Dosages
(general guidelines, many different dosage schedules)

Amantadine: 100 mg 1–2 times daily (up to 400 mg/day) PO

Carbidopa-levodopa: 10–25 mg carbidopa/100–250 mg levodopa 3–4 times daily PO, or 25 mg/100 mg or 50 mg/200 mg twice daily for extended release preparations PO

Entacapone: 200 mg up to 8 times daily PO

Pergolide: 50 mcg-1 mg/day 1–3 times daily (not to exceed 5 mg/day) PO

Pramipexole: 1.5–4.5 mg/day in 3 divided doses PO

Ropinirole: 0.25–1.5 mg/day 3 times daily (not to exceed 9 mg/day) PO

Selegiline: 10 mg in divided doses PO

Tolcapone: 100–200 mg 3 times daily PO

Administration

These drugs are usually given PO. Drugs are often started at low doses and then increased until optimal effectiveness is achieved. Effects may only be seen after 1 to 4 weeks of therapy, and chronic administration should not be stopped abruptly, because a severe Parkinsonian crisis may occur. Some drugs (e.g., levodopa) can produce an "on-off" syndrome, in which therapeutic effects might temporarily disappear (apomorphine is used to counteract the "off" episodes). After a while, some drugs lose effectiveness, which can sometimes be restored with "drug-free holidays." Some drugs are given concomitantly.

Contraindications

Contraindications include seizure disorders, and cardiac and psychiatric disorders.

Common Adverse Reactions

Adverse reactions include dizziness, sedation, drowsiness (with sleep attacks), hallucinations, involuntary movements, and hypotension. Malignant neuroleptic syndrome and rhabdomyolysis have been reported with entacapone.

Drug Interactions

- Drugs should not be used with MAO inhibitors; can increase the risk of hypotension with antihypertensives; and interact adversely with some antipsychotic drugs.

- Kava and vitamin B6 decrease the effectiveness of carbidopa-levodopa. Selegiline can interact with a large number of prescription and OTC drugs and can cause a hypertensive crisis when consuming tyramine-containing foods.

Implications for Physical Therapists

- Reinforce that patients on levodopa therapy should not take large doses of multivitamins or vitamin B_6 because these can reduce the drug's effectiveness.
- Patients on levodopa exhibiting the "off" phase during therapy should be rescheduled at times when they experience the "on" phase. Taking the medication with a light meal can often reduce the "off" phase.

- Be aware that patients on some of these drugs can show involuntary movements and dystonias, which should be reported to the treating physician.
- Some drugs can produce pronounced drowsiness with "sleep" attacks. Reschedule patient at different times after taking the drug if this is a problem.
- If a patient is taking entacapone and complains about muscle weakness or pain and brown-colored urine, notify a physician immediately because this could be a warning sign of rhabdomyolysis.
- Advise patients to change positions slowly because some drugs can cause marked orthostatic hypotension, which is particularly dangerous in these patients.

Corticosteroids

Common Drugs (selection of some of the most commonly used drugs)

Short-acting drugs
    Cortisone (Cortone)
    Hydrocortisone (Cortef, A-hydroCort, other)
Intermediate-acting drugs
    Methylprednisolone (A-methapred, Depoprep, Depoject, other)
    Prednisolone (Articulose, Cotolone, Predate, other)
    Prednisone (Cordrol, Deltasone, Orasone, other)
    Triamcinolone (Amcort, Aristocort, Clinacort, other)
Long-acting drugs
    Betamethasone (Celestone)
    Budesonide (Entocort)

Dexamethasone (Cortastat, Dalalone, Decadrol, Decameth, other)
Other

Indications

Corticosteroids are indicated in:

- *Inflammations* that are unwanted or excessive. An inflammation is characterized by swelling, redness, warmth, pain, and eventual tissue damage if they become excessive. The first three signs are initiated by vasodilation, allowing white blood cells to invade the tissue. This helps fight infections or helps heal damaged tissues. However, if an inflammation becomes excessive or is unwanted (autoimmune diseases, transplants, allergies, asthma, croup, rheumatoid arthritis, osteoarthritis, ankylosing spondylitis, bursitis, and other conditions), it starts to damage healthy tissue. Drugs are mostly analogues of natural hormones, which have a longer duration of action, possess more antiinflammatory activity (more therapeutic action), and have a lesser effect on metabolic processes (less adverse reactions). Drugs reduce or abolish unwanted or excessive inflammations in that they stabilize lysosomal membranes, preventing the release of proteolytic enzymes; decrease capillary permeability, inhibiting the migration of inflammatory white blood cells into tissues; affect lymph nodes, reducing antibody formation; and enhance the effects of circulating catecholamines like epinephrine, causing vasoconstriction.

- *Adrenocortical insufficiency*, when the adrenal glands do not produce enough glucocorticoids. Drugs are used as replacement therapy and supply glucocorticoid activity to the body.
- *Management of various skin, lung, ocular, and related inflammations.* Most uses are suppression or reduction of an excessive or unwanted inflammatory response.

Examples of Common Dosages
(general guidelines, many different dosage schedules)

Betamethasone: 0.6–7.2 mg once or in divided doses daily PO

Budesonide: 9 mg once daily PO
Cortisone: 25–300 mg once daily PO
Dexamethasone: 0.5–9 mg single or divided doses daily PO
Hydrocortisone: 20–240 mg 1–4 times daily PO
Methylprednisolone: 120–1180 mg 3–4 times daily PO
Prednisolone: 5–200 mg 1–4 times daily PO (depending on disease)
Prednisone: 5–200 mg 1–4 times daily PO (depending on disease)
Triamcinolone: 4–48 mg 1–4 times daily PO (depending on disease)

Administration

These drugs can be given IM, IV, rectally, topically, by inhalation, or PO. They differ depending on the route of administration in onset (1–2 hours) and duration (1–6 days). Drugs should not be discontinued abruptly because they suppress ACTH secretion, which needs time to recover and which, before recovery, can cause a glucocorticoid deficiency syndrome.

Contraindications

Corticosteroids should not be used during chronic infections, and live vaccines should not be administered during chronic high-dose therapy. They should be used with caution in children because the drugs retard growth.

Common Adverse Reactions

- Adverse reactions include either depression or euphoria, increased risk of infections, restlessness, anorexia, ecchymoses (blood-caused discolorations), petechiae (red spots), hypertension, osteoporosis, muscle wasting, weakening of tendons and ligaments, metabolic changes, fat shifts within the body ("buffalo hump", "moon face"), increased ocular pressure, and cataracts.

- Topically applied or inhaled drugs can cause the same side effects but on a milder scale (except cataract formation and increased ocular pressure after ocular use is enhanced, which will occur in some but not all patients).

Drug Interactions

- They can interact with a large number of drugs and might require increases in dosages of insulin and oral hypoglycemic agents, and enhance the effects of drugs that affect potassium excretion. They increase the risk of stomach ulcer with use of NSAIDs.
- Grapefruit juice can increase levels of some corticosteroids, leading to overdose effects.

Implications for Physical Therapists

- If you have an infection, wear a mask or do not handle patients who are on long-term, high-dose steroid therapy because their immune systems are weakened.
- If you notice signs such as "moon face" or "buffalo hump," notify or have patients notify a physician because the dosage might have to be adjusted.
- Be aware that older people on long-term, high-dose steroid therapy might have osteoporosis and might incur further weakening of bones. Exercise should be adjusted accordingly. However, gentle exercise can prevent or slow down osteoporosis.
- If you notice personality changes in your patient, notify or have the patient contact the physician because this can be a "steroid psychosis," and the drug or dose might have to be adjusted.
- If you notice muscle wasting, notify or have patients contact a physician, because steroids can interfere with muscle metabolism. However, gentle exercises can prevent or slow down this adverse process.
- Treat joints of patients who have received a steroid injection in a joint gently, because steroids can weaken ligaments and tendons.
- Measure blood pressure frequently, because these drugs can cause hypertension.

Diuretics

Common Drugs (selection of some of the most commonly used drugs)

Thiazide and thiazide-like diuretics
  Chlorothiazide (Diuril)
  Hydrochlorothiazide (Esidrix, Hydro-chlor, Microzide, other)
  Chlorthalidone (Hygroton, Thalitone)
  Indapamide (Lozol)
  Other
Loop diuretics
  Bumetanide (Bumex)
  Furosemide (Lasix)

Torsemide (Demadex)
Potassium-sparing diuretics
   Amiloride (Midamor)
   Spironolactone (Aldactone)
   Triamterene (Dyrenium)
Osmotic diuretics
   Mannitol (Osmitrol, Resectisol)

Indications

Diuretics are indicated in:

- *Hypertension*, in which they increase water and salt (sodium. potassium, other) excretion, and reduce blood volume and pressure. They possibly cause some sodium depletion in blood vessel walls, resulting in some vasodilatation that also reduces blood pressure.
- *Edema* or excessive fluid accumulation because of congestive heart failure or other causes, where they reduce this fluid accumulation by increasing water excretion.
- *Various problems* including attack of narrow-angle glaucoma to quickly reduce excessively elevated intraocular pressure, or cerebral edema (e.g., IV mannitol).

Examples of Common Dosages

(general guidelines, many different dosage schedules)

Chlorothiazide: 250–1000 mg/day as a single or divided doses PO
Hydrochlorothiazide: 12.5–100 mg/day in 1 or 2 doses up to 200 mg/day PO
Chlorthalidone: 25–100 mg/day once daily PO
Indapamide: 1.25–5 mg/day once PO

Bumetanide: 0.5–2 mg/day once with additional doses if needed up to 10 mg/day PO
Furosemide: 20–80 mg/day once or twice PO
Torsemide: 5–20 mg once daily PO
Amiloride: 5–10 mg/day PO (up to 20 mg)
Spironolactone: 12.5–400 mg/day as a single dose PO
Triamterene: 100 mg twice daily (not to exceed 300 mg/day) PO
Mannitol: 50–100 g as a 5%-25% solution IV

Administration

- Drugs can be given IV, IM, and PO. Drugs are often used in combination with each other or other drugs.
- Loop diuretics are the strongest diuretics but are also associated with more adverse reactions.

Contraindications

These drugs should not be given to patients with electrolyte imbalances. Thiazide diuretics may show cross-sensitivity with sulfonamides. Patients who show a tendency toward gout can have an increased risk of gout with thiazides because of hyperuricemia.

Common Adverse Reactions

Adverse reactions include dehydration (hypotension, tachycardia, dyspnea), hypokalemia (palpitations, skeletal muscle weakness or cramping, paralysis, nausea or vomiting, polydipsia, delirium, and depression) with thiazide and loop diuretics, and hyperkalemia (confusion, hyperexcitability, muscle weakness, flaccid paralysis, and arrhythmias) with the potassium-sparing diuretics. In addition, drugs can cause other electrolyte and metabolic imbalances (metabolic alkalosis), drowsiness, dizziness, orthostatic hypotension, and increases in blood glucose and cholesterol levels. Hearing loss (tinnitus) occurs mostly with loop diuretics after IV administration.

Drug Interactions

- Potassium-losing diuretics can cause severe hypokalemia with drugs that also cause potassium loss. Potassium loss increases digitalis toxicity and reduces lithium excretion precipitating lithium toxicity. Potassium-sparing diuretics can cause significant hyperkalemia in the presence of drugs such as ACE inhibitors, which also retain potassium. Hearing problems caused by loop diuretics are made worse by aminoglycosides.
- Licorice and herbal laxatives (senna) may increase the risk of hypokalemia. Ginkgo may decrease the antihypertensive effects.

Implications for Physical Therapists

- Advise patients to change position slowly, particularly when getting up, because drugs decrease blood pressure and carry the risk of orthostatic hypotension.
- Monitor patients for muscle activity and other unusual signs because some diuretics can cause hypokalemia, and others can cause hyperkalemia. If this is noticed, notify a physician immediately.
- UV light should be used with caution, and parts of the patient should be covered because some diuretics can cause photosensitivity reactions.
- When exercising patients in a warm environment, monitor sweating and recommend frequent water supplementation to prevent dehydration.

Drugs and Substance Abuse

This is only a short list of legal and illegal abused substances. A clear definition of dependence and addiction is given.

Alcohol

- Alcohol or ethanol is metabolized mostly by two enzymes at the rate of about 100 mg/kg/hr, or roughly 10 ml/hour/person (about one glass of wine or beer per hour in the average person). It is also partially exhaled by the lungs (thus the efficacy of breath-alyzer tests). It is evenly distributed throughout the body, and blood tests can predict tissue levels.
- Alcohol is a central nervous system depressant and seems to affect inhibitory pathways, first resulting usually in loss of inhibi-

tions and then resulting in aggressive behavior. This is followed by general CNS depression with impaired sensory function and muscular coordination; and changes in mood, personality, behavior, and mental activity. Intoxicated persons often are not aware of these impairments, and alcohol can cause the feeling of increased performance while there actually is a decrease.

- Small amounts of alcohol, such as one to two glasses of wine (in particular red wine) seem to be beneficial for maintaining good health, while large amounts consumed over long periods can lead to alcoholism, with significant health risks often exacerbated by poor diets and vitamin deficiencies (like lack of thiamine). Adverse reactions include damage to the liver (cirrhosis), stomach (ulcer), and heart and brain (e.g., Korsakoff/Wernicke syndrome, or memory loss and psychotic behavior), and in pregnant women can result in birth to children with fetal alcohol syndrome (facial/mental abnormalities).
- Alcoholism is treated, with limited success, with various drugs and behavioral modification techniques.
- Alcohol can enhance the sedative and gastric-damaging effects of many drugs.

Tobacco

- Tobacco smoke contains thousands of chemicals that the smoker inhales, of which nicotine, tar, and carbon monoxide (CO) are the most important.
- Nicotine will stimulate the nicotinic receptors in the brain, causing a rewarding feeling, and excessive smoking can lead to hypertension, tachycardia, gastric problems, and cardiovascular pathology.
- Tar is the product of incomplete combustion of organic material and causes inflammation of the lungs (smoker's cough, bronchitis, emphysema) and cancer of the throat, lungs, and bladder. If heavy smokers stop smoking, their chances of dying from cancer will slowly diminish.
- Carbon monoxide is also formed by incomplete combustion of tobacco and will bind to hemoglobin, replacing oxygen and leading to a reduction in the oxygen supply to all tissues (hemoglobin is converted to carboxyhemoglobin).
- Smoking cessation treatments include measured nicotine supply (gums, patches), drugs, and behavioral modification.

Marijuana

- Marijuana/hashish smoke contains many compounds, with tetrahydrocannabinol (THC) being the active, "rewarding" compound.
- Effects of THC include relaxation, disturbed sensory perception (interferes with driving a car), stimulation of appetite, and antiemetic (allowed in certain states for cancer patients to combat nausea and vomiting) effects.

- Chronic, heavy use might include the toxic effects of inhaled CO and tar (see Tobacco). The theory that marijuana is a stepping stone to other drugs has been largely abandoned.
- THC or dronabinol is available as a drug to reduce nausea and vomiting during cancer chemotherapy.

Heroin

- Heroin is converted in the body to morphine, which produces both CNS and peripheral effects (see *Opioid* or *Narcotic Analgesics*). Users tend to prefer heroin to morphine because heroin provides a quicker and more rewarding effect, crossing quickly into the brain.
- Methadone is used to treat heroin abuse and to prevent withdrawal symptoms.

Cocaine and Amphetamines

- Both drugs are sympathomimetic (see the sections on both Alpha and Beta Agonists) and stimulate adrenergic receptors. In the brain, they cause their "rewarding" effects mostly through the action of dopamine activity, whereas in the body, alpha and beta receptor stimulation prevail, with tachycardia and hypertension.
- Both drugs will counteract the therapeutic effects of alpha and beta blockers.

Dependence and Addiction

Physical dependence and addiction can occur with all drugs, be they these substances of abuse or prescription drugs.

- *Physical dependence* is an altered physiological state caused by the repeated administration of a drug or substance that later demands its continued use to prevent withdrawal or abstinence syndrome. The occurrence of withdrawal symptoms indicates the existence of physical dependence. Physical dependence carries certain health risks, but withdrawal can be dangerous or even life-threatening. The degree of physical dependence depends on the drug, dose, and length of use.
- *Withdrawal* occurs only after abrupt cessation of a drug or substance in a physically dependent individual. Signs and symptoms are usually opposite to original drug effects (for example, morphine, which can cause miosis and constipation; withdrawal causes mydriasis and diarrhea). For most drugs (illegal as well as legal), if medication is discontinued slowly (tapered off) after long-term, high-dose therapy, no withdrawal symptom should occur.
- *Addiction* is a behavioral pattern of compulsive drug or substance use characterized by the overwhelming involvement with the drug, the securing of its supply, and a high tendency to relapse after its cessation. Also, addiction can be described as "uncontrollable drug-using behavior," resulting in loss of "normal" functioning and harm to the user

and society. Controlled use of drugs is not considered addiction (e.g., social consumption of alcohol). Genetic and environmental factors seem to determine addiction to a large extent; some individuals can avoid or handle drugs or substances "socially" regardless of availability, whereas others cannot.

"Street Drug Toxicity"

- Illegally obtained drugs or substances carry additional risks in addition to those already associated with the substance, which can be more severe and even fatal because of illegal manufacturing and unscrupulous selling practices.
- The user can never be sure if the substance bought from street sellers is indeed the right drug (drugs that are sold on the street can often be more dangerous than what is "advertised"), is the right dose (often too high a dose is sold; this is responsible for most heroin-related deaths), or if it contains dangerous impurities (they can often be contaminated by chemicals that are much more toxic than the basic drug, such as rat poison, which can result in death). Furthermore, improper use carries significant health risks such as shared needles, which can spread hepatitis and AIDS.

Implications for Physical Therapists

- The physical therapist must be aware that many legal and illegal drugs can cause dependence, and that it is important for the patients to not stop these drugs abruptly, but to discontinue them slowly to avoid serious withdrawal reactions.
- The physical therapist must also be aware that addiction is associated not only with illegal drugs (although many users of such drugs are not addicted, but use them only occasionally) but also with excessive, long-term alcohol and tobacco use, and with excessive use of nasal sprays, androgenic steroids, or laxatives.
- The physical therapist can be helpful in advising the individual about the dangers of using or abusing certain substances and to encourage them to stop. This is particularly true when smoke or alcohol is detected on a patient's breath during therapy sessionss in the early part of the day.
- The physical therapist can warn illegal drug users—if known—or younger individuals who express thoughts about buying drugs on the street, that they may have serious ill effects and they could even die, not only from the substances, but also from their unsanitary and unprofessional manufacturing techniques and unscrupulous selling practices.

Drugs and Blood Clotting

Common Drugs (Selection of some of the Most Commonly Used Drugs)

Oral anticoagulants
  Warfarin (Coumadin)
Parental anticoagulants
  Heparin (Fragmin, Lovenox, Arixtra, Innohep)
  Other
Antiplatelet drugs
  Aspirin
  Clopidogrel (Plavix)
  Dipyridamole (Dipridacot)
Fibrinolytic or thrombolytic drugs
  Alteplase (TPA) or Activase
  Reteplase
  Streptokinase
  Urokinase
Clotting factors
  Factors VIII and IX

Indications

Drugs for blood clotting are indicated in:

- *Pulmonary embolism*, when an artery in the lung becomes blocked. In most cases, the blockage is caused by one or more blood clots that travel to the lungs from another part of the body. It manifests itself with sudden shortness of breath, chest pain often mimicking a heart attack, cough, tachycardia, wheezing, leg swelling, sweating, anxiety, and lightheadedness or fainting. It is mostly mild but can become fatal. Anticoagulants prevent formation of thrombi by interfering with the synthesis of vitamin K–dependent clotting factors (warfarin) or by inhibiting thrombin formation (heparin, which is a natural product).

- *Strokes* occur mostly when the blood supply to a part of the brain is reduced or stopped by a blood clot (ischemic stroke) so that within a few minutes neurons start to die. Warning signs include trouble with walking, dizziness, loss of balance or coordination, numbness, trouble speaking or seeing, and persistent headache. If signs are fleeting, it is called a transient ischemic attack, in which blood flow is only temporarily interrupted. The signs and symptoms are similar but usually milder and disappear mostly within minutes, but they should be brought to the attention of a physician. A few strokes are caused by bleeding in the brain (hemorrhagic strokes). Intervention of a stroke must occur quickly to prevent brain damage. It is recommended not to give aspirin at home but to rush the individual to a hospital as soon as possible. It will then be determined what type of stroke it is. If it is a hemorrhagic stroke, surgery might be indicated (administration of aspirin would have increased further bleeding). In the case of an ischemic stroke, aspirin is given, followed by fibrinolytic drugs to dissolve the clot. Aspirin prevents platelet aggregation by interfering with thromboxane formation necessary for platelet aggregation, and fibrinolytic drugs dissolve unwanted blood clots usually by activating plasmin formation. Fibrinolytic drugs must be administered within 3 hours, although recently it has been shown that they may still work after this time.

- *Heart attack* or myocardial infarction can occur when a blood clot blocks a coronary blood vessel and prevents blood flow and supply of nutrients and oxygen to cardiac muscle, resulting in damage and death of cardiac tissue. Common signs and symptoms of a heart attack include pressure and pain in the center of the chest that extends to the shoulder, arm, back, or teeth and jaw; shortness of breath; sweating; fainting; and nausea and vomiting. Aspirin and clopidogrel can be given. The latter reduces ATP attachment to platelets and decreases platelet aggregation.

- *Atrial fibrillation or prosthetic heart valves*, which can give rise to the formation of thrombi. These can later travel and block blood vessels leading to tissue damage. Drugs reduce their formation and prevent possible tissue damage. Clopidogrel is sometimes used.

- *Deep vein thrombosis prevention*, in which these drugs dissolve or prevent the formation of thrombi and their possible travel through the vascular system.

- *Hemophilia* is a rare, inherited bleeding disorder in which blood does not clot normally. Bleeding episodes can range from mild to fatal and can be caused by injuries or can be internal. The cause is a lack of certain clotting factors. Hemophilia A is caused by a lack of or too little clotting factor VIII, and hemophilia B is caused by low levels of clotting factor IX. Treatment involves replacement therapy by giving or replacing the necessary clotting factor. These factors can be obtained from human blood or be made by recombinant techniques. They are injected.

Examples of Common Dosages
(general guidelines, many different dosage schedules)

Warfarin: 2.5–10 mg/day PO or IV
Heparin: Depending on the preparation SC
Aspirin: 81 mg once daily PO
Clopidogrel: 75 mg once daily PO
Dipyridamole: 225–400 mg in 3–4 divided doses daily PO

Administration

These drugs can be given IV, SC, or PO. A number of drugs in the previous categories are usually only administered in the hospital (fibrinolytic or thrombolytic drugs).

Contraindications

Contraindications or cautious use include patients for risk of bleeding and pending surgery, in which case drugs should be stopped about 1 week before.

Common Adverse Reactions

Adverse reactions include fatigue, headache, increased risk of bleeding by external or internal injuries, and, rarely, a potentially fatal thrombotic thrombocytic purpura. Orthostatic hypotension can occur with dipyridamole. Discontinuation of long-term therapy with these drugs, such as before surgery, can carry a slightly increased risk of the formation of thrombi.

Drug Interactions
- They can interact with NSAIDs by increasing bleeding episodes.
- Risk of bleeding is increased with concurrent use of ginkgo, garlic, ginseng, and other herbal products. Foods high in vitamin K content may antagonize the action of warfarin.

Implications for Physical Therapists
- If patients complain about nose bleeds, bleeding gums, unusual bruising, or black stools, notify or have patient contact a physician because this might require a dose adjustment.
- Hold older, frail people on these medications gently because firm or tight handling can lead to bruising or bleeding episodes.
- Advise patients not to take over-the-counter NSAIDs, or to notify physician before taking these drugs, because they can increase the risk of bleeding.
- Patients should use vitamins only with the advice of a physician. In particular, they should avoid vitamin K preparations when on anticoagulant therapy.
- Instruct patients to strictly adhere to the dosing schedule because doses taken too rapidly or in excess can increase the risk of severe bleeding.
- Advise older patients who do not take these medications not to sit quietly for too long, or to periodically get up, tense their legs, or walk, e.g., on long airplane flights, to exercise leg muscles, keep blood flowing, and prevent thrombi formation. Pressure stockings (TED hose) can also be used.

Drugs and Bone
Common Drugs (selection of some of the most commonly used drugs)
Calcium supplements
　　Many different preparations with or without vitamin D supplementation
Bisphosphonates
　　Alendronate (Fosamax)
　　Etidronate (Didronel)
　　Ibandronate (Boniva)
　　Pamidronate (Aredia)
　　Risedronate (Actonel)
Calcitonin
　　Calcitonin (Calcimar, Salmonine, other)
Parathyroid hormone
　　Teriparatide (Forteo)

Indications
Drugs are indicated in:
- *Osteoporosis*, characterized by excessive porosity of the bone caused by enlargement of the canals or formation of cavities.

This can lead to bone fractures. All drugs slow down the progression of the disease by promoting new and stronger bone formation. Bone formation can be increased by supplying calcium, which might be missing in the diet or is not absorbed fully. Calcium in supplements is mostly combined with carbonate, citrate, phosphate, lactate, and gluconate. Vitamin D supplementation will increase calcium absorption. Bisphosphonates, which seem to be incorporated into bone, reduce bone destruction and seem to promote a more adequate and efficient mineralization. Calcitonin will also increase bone formation.

- Drugs also counteract steroid-induced osteoporosis. In severe cases, a synthetic parathyroid hormone preparation can be injected.
- *Hypoparathyroidism*, which leads to impaired bone breakdown and hypocalcemia. Calcium and vitamin D supply the needed calcium for the body, or injection of the parathyroid hormone preparation can be administered.
- *Rickets*, which is a vitamin D deficiency in children (not usually seen anymore in this country but evident in other parts of the world) that causes abnormal bone formation. Calcium and vitamin D supply the needed calcium for the body.
- Other uses include *certain cancers*, *osteomalacia*, and *Paget disease*.

Examples of Common Dosages
(general guidelines, many different dosage schedules)

Calcium supplements

Alendronate: 10 mg once daily or 70 mg once weekly PO

Etidronate: 5–10 mg/kg/day once daily PO

Ibandronate: 2.5 mg once daily or 150 mg once a month PO

Pamidronate: 30–90 mg in single or divided doses IV

Risedronate: 5 mg once daily or 35 mg once weekly PO

Calcitonin: 200 IU/day by nasal spray

Teriparatide: 20 mcg/day SC

Administration

Bisphosphonates must be taken PO with water on an empty stomach in the morning while sitting or standing for at least 30 to 60 minutes (to prevent reflux into esophagus, which can cause severe irritations). The parathyroid hormone preparation is injected.

Contraindications

Bisphosphonates should not be used by patients with renal and GI disorders.

Common Adverse Reactions

Bisphosphonates are generally well tolerated except for some GI distress, particularly if NSAIDs are being used. Calcitonin can cause some allergic reactions. The parathyroid hormone preparation may cause pain at the site of the injection, some weakness, and, still uncertain, may increase the risk of bone cancer.

Drug Interactions

Bisphosphonates should not be taken with caffeine drinks or mineral water.

Implications for Physical Therapists

- Encourage the patient to use a balanced diet; to walk at least an hour a day in daylight; and to do weight-bearing exercises to strengthen bones and to avoid possible fractures. Furthermore, the patient at risk should stop smoking and avoid excessive alcohol consumption.
- Advise patients to follow administration schedule for the bisphosphonates exactly as prescribed because significant adverse reactions can otherwise occur.

Drugs and the Thyroid Gland

Common Drugs (selection of some of the most commonly used drugs)

Hypothyroidism
  Liothyronine (T3) (Cytomel, Triostat, other)
  Levothyroxine (T4) (Synthroid, Levo-T, other)
Hyperthyroidism
  Propylthiouracil (Propylthiouracil)
  Other

Indications

Drugs for the thyroid gland are indicated in:

- *Hypothyroidism*, or a lack of sufficient hormone secretion, which can be caused by an autoimmune disease but can also result from the surgical removal of a cancerous gland. It manifests itself as physical and mental fatigue, weight gain, dry and rough skin, and muscle cramps and aches. Drug therapy consists of replacement therapy with hormones. Both thyroxine and liothyronine have a somewhat delayed onset of action, and levothyroxine is preferred for long-term therapy. Drugs have a narrow margin of safety, and it is often difficult to find and maintain the right dose.
- *Hyperthyroidism*, or a surplus of the hormone, which can also be caused by an autoimmune disease where antibodies stimulate the gland to produce too much hormone. It manifests itself in palpitations and tachycardia, heat intolerance, insomnia, weight loss, warm and moist skin, and muscle weakness. Propylthiouracil and related drugs will inhibit the organification of iodide and reduce excessive levels of the hormone. Other treatments are hospital procedures such as surgery or destruction of glandular tissue with radioactive iodide.

Examples of Common Dosages (general guidelines, many different dosage schedules)

Liothyronine: 25–75 mcg /day PO
Levothyroxine: 50–200 mcg/day PO
Propylthiouracil: 100–300 mg 3 times daily PO

Administration

Hormones and drugs are taken PO.

Contraindications

Hormones are contraindicated (or should be used with caution) in patients with adrenal insufficiency and myocardial infarctions; and propylthiouracil is contraindicated (or should be used with caution) in patients with hepatic diseases and bone marrow depression.

Common Adverse Reactions

Generally, adverse reactions of hormone replacement therapy often result from overdosing and include nervousness and excitability, tachycardia, palpitations, weight loss, heat intolerance, and angina in compromised patients. Propylthiouracil may cause hepatic and renal problems, as well as agranulocytosis, bleeding episodes, and hypothyroidism if doses are too high.

Drug Interactions

- Thyroid hormones increase the effects of anticoagulants and decrease effectiveness of insulin and oral hypoglycemics. Propylthiouracil interacts with iodide and lithium.
- Efficacy of thyroid hormones is decreased by soy, bugleweed, and carnitine. Also, foods high in iodine should be avoided.

Implications for Physical Therapists

- Observe patients on hormone replacement therapy carefully and check for signs and symptoms of hyper- or hypothyroidism. If present, contact or ask patients to contact a physician because this might indicate a dose adjustment.
- Advise patients on hormone replacement therapy who lose weight and show nervousness and excitability if they follow the physician's instructions or take too much, because hormones are not to be used for losing weight.
- Patients on propylthiouracil should be watched for yellowing skin and eyes, indicating jaundice, bleeding episodes; and an unexplained sore throat, indicating agranulocytosis. If these occur, contact or have patients inform a physician about these observations.
- If a patient on propylthiouracil starts to show hypothyroidism, contact or have patient contact a physician because this might necessitate a reduction in dose.

Female Hormones

Common Drugs (selection of some of the most commonly used drugs)

Estrogens
  Estradiol (Estrace, Vivelle, other)
  Ethinyl (Estradiol Estinyl)
  Other
Progestins
  Progesterone (Gesterol, Prometrium)
  Norgestrel (Ovrette)
  Other
Contraceptives
  Ethinyl estradiol
  plus desogestrel (Desogen, Mircette, other)
  ethynodiol (Demulen, Zovia)
  Levonorgestrel (Levlen, Nordette, other)
  Norethindrone (Loestrin, Brevicon, other)
  Norgestimate (Ortho-Cyclen, other)
  Norgestrel (Ovral)
  Mestranol
  plus norethindrone (Genora, Norinyl, other)
  Norethindrone (Micronor)
  Norgestrel (Ovrette)
  Other
Postcoital drugs
  Mifepristone (Mifeprex)
  Other
Estrogen receptor modulators
  Raloxifene (Evista)
  Tamoxifen (Nolvadex)
  Other

Indications

Female hormones are indicated in:

- *Estrogen replacement therapy*, where an estrogen deficiency causes postmenopausal problems (hot flashes, bone loss, vaginal dystrophy). Exogenous estrogen will now assume the role of the deficient endogenous hormones and reduce these problems. This practice is now reserved for severe cases only.
- *Amenorrhea and dysfunctional uterine bleeding* caused by an abnormal hormone balance. Estrogens and/or progestins can restore the normal balance.
- *Contraception.* The combination pill estrogen plus progesterone delivers high levels of both hormones into the body, suppressing follicle-stimulating hormone (FSH) and luteinizing hormone (LH) secretion from the pituitary gland and preventing the start of a new cycle of ovulation ("pseudo-pregnancy"). This pill is 99% to 100% effective. In addition, progesterone causes a vaginal sperm-hostile environment, preventing sperm from traveling further. The progesterone-only pill works mostly by the creation of the sperm-hostile environment and also by somewhat reducing FSH and LH secretion. Its effectiveness is about 98%. Lately, newer contraceptive schedules have been introduced that cause a 3-month or longer cycle.
- *Postcoital intervention*, when no conception was intended after unprotected sex. High doses of estrogens and/or progesterone are given (within days) and prob-

ably act by inhibiting implantation of the fertilized egg. Similarly, mifepristone (taken within 50 days) blocks the progesterone receptors in the uterus, which support the endometrium and leads to endometrial shedding (sometimes followed by administration of a prostaglandin analogue, misoprostol, which stimulates uterine contractions and helps in this process).

- *Breast cancer*, which in some women is promoted by estrogen receptor activity. Estrogen receptor blockers or modulators will block these receptors and reduce estrogen's cancer-promoting effects.
- Other uses include treatment of *endometriosis*, *prostate cancer*, and *endometrial cancer*.

Examples of Common Dosages
(general guidelines, many different dosage schedules)

Estradiol: 1–2 mg/day PO
Ethinyl Estradiol: 0.02 mg or 0.05 mg daily PO
Contraceptives: Many different combinations and dosages
Mifepristone: 600 mg in 3 divided doses PO (followed by 400 mg misoprostol PO)
Raloxifene: 60 mg once daily PO
Tamoxifen: 10–20 mg 2 times daily PO

Administration

- Depending on the drug, they can be given orally, IM, SC, by spray, patch, implant, or vaginal ring. The contraceptive combination pill is either given for 3 weeks with 1 week of placebos (1-month cycle) or for 84 days with 1 week of placebos (3-month cycle).
- It is important to take contraceptives as directed because breakthrough bleeding and reduced protection can occur. General guidelines (will vary among drugs) are: If one dose is missed and remembered the same day, then the missed dose should be taken immediately. If it is remembered the next day, two tablets are taken on that day and then back to one tablet per day. If two doses are missed, two tablets are taken for two days, then return to one tablet per day. If three or more tablets are missed, consult a physician, pharmacist, or nurse.

Contraindications

These drugs should not be used in patients with thromboembolic disorders.

Common Adverse Reactions

Estrogen replacement therapy has been associated with a higher risk of myocardial infarctions, stroke, pulmonary embolism, and thromboembolism, and can increase the risk of endometrial and breast cancer, although the latter is restricted to a subset of women. Both hormones can cause sodium and water retention with weight gain and swelling of the feet. Estrogens in susceptible individuals might cause depression. Contraceptives carry the same risks and smoking intensifies the blood-clotting effects. Tamoxifen has been associated with uterine malignancies.

Drug Interactions

These drugs can interact with a number of other drugs. Estrogens are contraindicated with tamoxifen, raloxifene, and steroids. Saw palmetto decreases their effectiveness.

Implications for Physical Therapists

- Patients on estrogens and in particular on contraceptives should be advised to stop smoking if they do. Explain the increased risk of cardiovascular accidents with this habit.
- If a patient complains about unexplainable pain in the legs, notify or have patient contact the physician immediately because this could indicate a deep vein thrombosis, which needs quick attention to prevent life-threatening problems.
- Check blood pressure periodically because salt retention in susceptible individuals can cause hypertension.
- If you notice that a patient on estrogens is fatigued and depressed, have patient notify physician because estrogens can cause depression.
- Inform patients that it is important to take contraceptives as directed because missed doses reduce or negate protection.
- Inform patients that contraceptives protect against pregnancy but not venereal diseases. Only condoms do this.

Gastrointestinal Drugs

Common Drugs (selection of some of the most commonly used drugs)

Antacids
H2 blockers
    Cimetidine (Tagamet)
    Famotidine (Pepcid)
    Nizatidine (Axid)
    Ranitidine (Zantac)
Proton pump inhibitors
    Esomeprazole (Nexium)
    Lansoprazole (Prevacid)
    Omeprazole (Prilosec)
    Pantoprazole (Protonix)
    Rabeprazole (Aciphex)
Antidiarrheal drugs
    Kaolin/pectin (Kapectolin)
    Bismuth (Pepto-Bismol)
    Diphenoxylate (Lomotil, Lonox, other)
    Loperamide (Imodium, other)
    Other
Laxatives
    Psyllium (Metamucil)
    Bisacodyl (Dulcolax, Deficol, Correctol)
    Senna (Senokot, Other)
    Docusate (Colace, Sulfolax, Other)
    Other

Indications

Gastrointestinal drugs are indicated in:

- *Dyspepsia, gastritis, and peptic ulcer,* where excessive acid production (among other causes such as bacteria) irritates and finally erodes the mucosa, causing an ulcer. Drugs reduce acid formation and inflammations and promote healing of ulcers. Antacids consist of a base such as carbonate, silicate, or hydroxide, which is combined with aluminum, calcium, or magnesium. The antacids combine with the acid and remove H+. The H2 blockers block the action of histamine on H2 receptors, and the proton pump inhibitors inhibit the H+ pump, which in both cases leads to a reduction in H+ secretion.

- *Gastroesophageal reflux disease* (GERD), where acid enters the esophagus causing inflammation, pain, spasm, and possibly cancer. Drugs reduce acid production so that less or no acid will enter the esophagus.

- *Constipation*, where peristalsis is decreased, which can lead to fecal impacts. Drugs increase peristalsis and promote fecal transport and evacuation. The laxatives increase the bulk in the intestines, promoting the stretch reflex (psyllium), soften the stool (docusate), or irritate the intestines (bisacodyl, senna), resulting in all cases in increased peristalsis and easier defecation.

- *Diarrhea*, where excessive motility leads to frequent evacuations that can result in marked water and electrolyte losses. Drugs slow peristalsis and reduce or prevent fluid and electrolyte loss. Antidiarrheal drugs such as the absorbents (kaolin/pectin, bismuth) absorb substances that might increase peristalsis, and diphenoxylate and loperamide reduce

intestinal muscle activity, which reduces peristalsis.

Examples of Common Dosages
(general guidelines, many different dosage schedules)

Cimetidine: 300–1600 mg/day in divided doses PO

Famotidine: 20–40 mg/day once daily PO

Nizatidine: 150 mg 1–2 times daily PO

Ranitidine: 150 mg 1–2 times daily PO

Esomeprazole: 20–40 mg/day once daily PO

Lansoprazole: 15–30 mg/day once daily PO

Omeprazole: 20–40 mg/day once daily PO

Pantoprazole: 40 mg/day once daily PO

Rabeprazole: 20 mg/day once daily PO

Kaolin/pectin: 60–120 ml after loose bowel movement PO

Bismuth: 525–1050 mg several times as needed PO

Diphenoxylate: 5 mg 3 times daily (combined with atropine) PO

Loperamide: 4 mg followed by 2 mg up to 16 mg/day PO

Psyllium: 1–2 tsp in 8 oz water 2–3 times daily PO

Bisacodyl: 10–30 mg 1–2 times daily PO

Docusate: 50–300 once daily PO

Senna: 1–8 tabs/day PO

Administration
Most drugs are given PO, with some also available rectally.

Contraindications

These drugs should not be used or must be used with caution in patients with a number of problems, depending on the drug employed.

Common Adverse Reactions

Adverse reactions differ among drugs. A rebound phenomenon (increased H+ secretion) can occur after long-term use of acid reducers. Large doses of antacids cause constipation (aluminum) or diarrhea (magnesium). H2 blockers can cause some dizziness and, rarely, blood disorders. Proton pump inhibitors show few adverse reactions, although some might, rarely, cause blood disorders and Stevens-Johnson syndrome. Loperamide and diphenoxylate may cause nausea, drowsiness, and dizziness. Irritating laxatives may cause nausea and intestinal cramps. Long-term use can lead to laxative dependence, in which physiological functions of the intestines start to decline.

Drug Interactions

Interactions with other drugs depend on the individual drug. Antacids reduce the availability of some antibiotics from the intestines. Altering the pH of the stomach can affect solubility and absorption of certain medications. Observe instructions.

Implications for Physical Therapists

- Instruct patients who take OTC cimetidine to do so not for more than 2 weeks or to consult a physician if further use is needed.
- Instruct patients that OTC preparations should be taken only exactly as indicated on packages and only for a short period of time. If no relief is obtained, a physician must be consulted because there could be more serious underlying problems.
- Inform patients that proper eating habits with the consumption of bulk (i.e., fiber) can reduce constipation problems.
- Advise patients against long-term use of laxatives—unless prescribed by a physician—because this could lead to laxative dependence. Tell patients that individuals differ in their bowel movements and that a bowel movement must not occur every day.

Hemopoietics

Common Drugs (selection of some of the most commonly used drugs)

Iron preparations (Feosol, Feostat, Feratab, Ferrlecit, other)
Epoetin (Epogen, Procrit)
Nandrolone (Deca-Durabolin, Kabolin)

Cyanocobalamin (Cobex, Cobolin-M, Nascobal, Vibal, other)
Hydroxocobalamin (Alphamin, Vibal LA, other)
Folic acid (Apo-Folic, Folate, Folvite, other)

Indications

Hemopoietic drugs are indicated in:

- *Iron-deficiency anemia* (extensive blood loss, severe menstruation, kidney problems requiring hemodialysis). Iron is part of hemoglobin and necessary for oxygen transport. Supplemental iron is available in different combinations, with an onset of about 4 days and peak effects at 1–2 weeks.
- *Folic acid deficiency anemia*. Folic acid is necessary for the synthesis of hemoglobin. Therapy consists of supplying missing folic acid.
- *B_{12} deficiency or pernicious anemia* (mostly caused by a lack of intrinsic factor, which promotes B_{12} absorption). Pernicious anemia also damages the nervous system. B_{12} is also necessary for hemoglobin synthesis. This anemia is treated with cyanocobalamin and hydroxocobalamin.
- Anemias caused by *chemotherapy or renal failure* are treated with epoetin and/or nandrolone. Epoetin stimulates erythrocyte formation, and nandrolone stimulates endogenous erythropoietin synthesis.

Common Dosages (general guidelines, many different dosage schedules)

Ferrous preparations: 120–240 mg/day in 2–4 divided doses PO

Iron polysaccharide: 50–100 mg/day twice daily as tablets or 150–300 mg/day as capsules PO

Epoetin: 50–100 units/kg 3 times weekly SC/IV

Nandrolone: 50–100 mg q week IM

Folic acid: 1 mg/day initially, then 0.5 mg daily PO

Cyanocobalamin: 1000 mcg daily PO or 500 mcg weekly by nasal spray or 30–100 mcg/day IM

Administration

These drugs can be given PO, IM, SC, IV, or via nasal spray. Onset of action is delayed and varies among medications and routes of administration.

Contraindications

Iron preparations should be used with extreme caution in patients with GI problems (ulcer).

Common Adverse Reactions

Iron preparations can cause GI problems (epigastric pain, constipation) and color stool black (masking GI bleeding). Overdosing leads to iron toxicity (bluish lips, drowsiness, weakness, seizures). Epoetin can cause hypertension, and nandrolone can cause allergic reactions. Folic acid and B_{12} are relatively safe.

Drug Interactions

Iron preparations chelate with tetracyclines and quinolones, and reduce their absorption. Vitamin C increases and food decreases iron absorption.

Implications for Physical Therapists

- If a patient is exhausted easily and appears bluish and anemic, advise them to see a physician and warn against self-medication, because different types of anemia exist and require special therapies.

Brittle, concave nails with ridges often indicate an iron deficiency anemia.

- Warn patients who use iron or folic acid without medical advice to treat an anemic condition to consult a physician, because a B_{12}-deficient anemia may respond somewhat to these preparations but nerve damage can continue unchecked.
- If a patient is using iron preparations and has black stools but also severe epigastric pain, advise the patient to see a physician, because this could indicate internal bleeding. Also advise the patient not to overdose with iron because this can lead to iron toxicity.
- Advise pregnant patients if not already recommended by physician to supplement with folic acid, even in the absence of an anemic condition, to reduce the risk of fetal abnormalities (spina bifida).

Hypoglycemics I

Common Drugs (selection of some of the most commonly used drugs)

Insulin lispro/protamine insulin (Humalog 75/25)

NPH/regular insulin mixtures (Humulin 50/50, 70/30, Novolin 70/30)

Short-acting insulin (Humulin R, Novolin R)

Intermediate-acting insulins

Isophane insulin (Humulin N, NPHIletin II)

Lente (zinc) insulin (Humulin L, Novolin ge Lente)

Long-acting insulins

Ultralente (zinc) insulin (Humulin U Ultralente, Novolin U)

Insulin glargine (Lantus)

Rapid-acting insulins

Insulin aspart (NovoLog)

Insulin lispro (Humalog)

Insulin glulisine (Apidra)

Indications

These drugs are indicated in:

- *Diabetes mellitus*, which is caused by a deficiency or lack of the pancreatic hormone insulin, which regulates blood glucose levels. It manifests itself as polydipsia and polyuria, with highly increased blood glucose levels (spilling into the urine), leading if left untreated to ocular, renal, and cardiovascular health consequences, as well as ketoacidosis. It can be divided into two types. Type 1 can be caused by an autoimmune or viral disease in which the insulin-producing beta cells in the pancreas are destroyed or nonfunctioning. Type 2 usually is an adult-onset condition, often caused by genetic factors as well as obesity. In this case there is either an insufficient release of insulin from the pancreas or unresponsive insulin receptors on tissues.

Insulin is injected (because oral preparations would be destroyed in the stomach) in type 1 to replace the missing endogenous hormone. In type 2, treatment starts with carbohydrate restrictions, exercise, and weight loss, and if unsuccessful, is followed by oral hypoglycemics (see Hypoglycemic Drugs II) and later insulin.

- *Diabetic ketoacidosis*, in which organic acids and ketone bodies are formed from fat because of poor glucose control, which can be life-threatening. Short-acting insulins plus other drugs and measures are used to restore homeostasis.

Examples of Common Dosages
(general guidelines, many different dosage schedules)

Insulin lispro/protamine insulin: 0.5–1 unit/kg/day

NPH/regular insulin mixtures: 0.5–1 unit/kg/day

Short-acting insulin: 0.5–1 unit/kg/hr

Intermediate-acting insulins: 0.5–1 unit/kg/day

Long-acting insulins: 0.5–1 unit/kg/day.

Rapid-acting insulins: 0.5–1 unit/kg/day

Administration

- Insulin has to be injected SC (IV for ketoacidosis) or given by pump or nasally. It now comes mostly from human recombinant DNA sources. Preparations are manufactured to have different onsets and durations of action to suit the characteristics of the disease of the individual patient. Onset of action ranges from 15 to 60 minutes and duration of action from 2 to 24 hours. Some preparations are used in the morning and others before meals.

- Stress, exercise, trauma, infections, or changes in diet may change the glucose response to insulin and might require dosage adjustments.

Contraindications

There are no major contraindications, except that nasal preparations should not be used in cases of lung problems like asthma or emphysema.

Common Adverse Reactions

The most common adverse reactions are hypersensitivity reactions, which can range from rashes and itching to an anaphylactic reaction. Hyperglycemia and hypoglycemia (sweating, weakness, dizziness, tremor, tachycardia, and unconsciousness) can result from too little or too much insulin. Insulin can cause local lipoatrophy or lipohypertrophy, which can be minimized by changing injection sites. Poorly controlled glucose levels can lead to ketoacidosis (fatigue, flushed skin, nausea, vomiting, and dyspnea) that can be life-threatening.

Drug Interactions

- Glucose-lowering effects may be reduced by a large number of drugs including corticosteroids, certain antipsychotic and antiviral drugs, and diuretics. Glucose-lowering effects may be enhanced by ACE inhibitors and salicylates. Beta blockers may mask the onset of a hypoglycemic reaction.

- Glucosamine, chromium, and coenzyme Q10 enhance blood glucose levels, lowering the effects of insulin.

Implications for Physical Therapists

- Make sure that the patient wears an identification tag indicating that he or she is a diabetic and what type and dose of insulin is being used. Also, make sure that the patient carries some sugar, a glucose preparation, or sweetened orange juice to counteract a possible hypoglycemic reaction.
- Do not recommend glucosamine to diabetic patients to treat joint problems unless this has been cleared with a physician, because glucosamine can cause hypoglycemic episodes in unadjusted insulin dosages.
- Be aware of the occurrence of hypoglycemia as well as hyperglycemia (unusual thirst, drowsiness, fruit-like breath, flushed). Treat the first with sugar (artificial sweeteners do not work) and the other by asking the patient to administer the needed insulin injection.
- Do not massage the site of injection because this could cause an unwanted increase in insulin absorption and a hypoglycemic reaction.
- Exercise a diabetic patient carefully, especially at the beginning of insulin therapy, because exercise can reduce blood glucose levels. Also suggest having insulin injected into the abdomen instead of skeletal muscle. Check glucose levels during and after exercise.

Hypoglycemics II

Common Drugs (selection of some of the most commonly used drugs)

Glucosidase inhibitors
    Acarbose (Precose)
    Miglitol (Glyset)
Biguanides
    Metformin (Fortamet, Glucophage, Riomet)
Meglitinides
    Nateglinide (Starlix)
    Repaglinide (GlucoNorm, Prandin)
    Sulfonylureas
    Glimepiride (Amaryl)
    Glipizide (Glucotrol)
    Glyburide (Diabeta, Glynase, Micronase)
Thiazolidinediones
    Pioglitazone (Actos)
    Rosiglitazone (Avandia)

Hormones
    Pramlintide (Symlin)
Insulin release facilitators
    Exenatide (Byetta)
    Sitagliptin (Januvia)

Indications

These drugs are indicated in:

Diabetes mellitus, which is caused by a deficiency or lack of the pancreatic hormone insulin, which regulates blood glucose levels. It manifests itself as polydipsia and polyuria with highly increased blood glucose levels (spilling into the urine), leading if left untreated to ocular, renal, and cardiovascular health consequences, as well as ketoacidosis. It can be divided into two types. Type 1 can be caused by an autoimmune or viral disease in which the insulin-producing beta cells in the pancreas are destroyed or nonfunctioning. Type 2 usually is an adult-onset condition often caused by genetic factors as well as obesity. In this case there is either an insufficient release of insulin from the pancreas or unresponsive insulin receptors on tissues.

Drugs used in the treatment of type 2 diabetes mellitus vary among patients. Treatment usually starts with carbohydrate restrictions, exercise, and weight loss.

Drugs work by different mechanisms to lower elevated blood glucose. Glucosidase inhibitors lower postprandial blood glucose by inhibiting alpha-glucosidase in the GI tract, which is involved in the breakdown of carbohydrates and reduces sugar absorption. Biguanides decrease hepatic glucose production, somewhat reduce intestinal glucose absorption, and increase insulin sensitivity. Meglitinides close pancreatic potassium channels and open calcium channels, which causes insulin release. Sulfonylureas release insulin from the pancreas, may increase insulin receptor sensitivity, and decrease hepatic glucose formation. Thiazolidinediones act as agonists on cellular insulin receptors and improve glucose uptake into tissues. Pramlintide slows gastric emptying, decreases glucagon secretion, and curbs appetite to reduce postprandial hyperglycemia. Insulin-release facilitators mimic the action of endogenous compounds, which facilitates insulin release.

If drugs do not provide adequate glucose control, insulin has to be used (see Hypoglycemic Drugs I).

Examples of Common Dosages
(general guidelines, many different dosage schedules)

Acarbose: 50–100 mg 3 times daily PO

Miglitol: 25–100 mg 3 times daily PO

Metformin: 500 mg 2 times daily up to 2000 mg/day PO, or 500–1000 mg once daily up to 2500 mg as extended release tablets PO

Nateglinide: 120 mg 3 times daily PO

Repaglinide: 0.5–4 mg 3 times daily not to exceed 16 mg/day PO

Glimepiride: 1–2 mg once daily to be increased to 8 mg/day PO

Glipizide: 2.5–40 mg/day PO

Glyburide: 1.25–20 mg once daily PO or 1.5–12 mg 2 times daily PO as micronized preparation

Pioglitazone: 15–45 mg once a day PO

Rosiglitazone: 4–8 mg once or 2–4 mg twice a day PO

Sitagliptin: 25–200 mg once daily PO

Pramlintide: 60–120 mcg once daily SC

Administration

Hypoglycemic drugs are given PO and SC (using a pen). Some orally administered drugs may take time to become fully effective. Hypoglycemic drugs may be used in combination with each other or with insulin.

Contraindications

These drugs should not be used in or used with caution in patients with hepatic failure.

Common Adverse Reactions

Hypoglycemic drugs can cause hypoglycemia (sweating, weakness, dizziness, tremor, tachycardia, and unconsciousness), but this occurs least with glucosidase inhibitors, thiazolidinediones, and biguanides. Drugs can cause nausea and GI problems. Glucosidase inhibitors also cause flatulence. Biguanides can cause lactic acidosis (chills, dizziness, hypotension, muscle pain, bradycardia, and dyspnea), which can be serious. Sulfonylureas cause photosensitization and rarely, agranulocytosis and aplastic anemia. Rosiglitazone may increase the risk of cardiovascular problems such as congestive heart failure (early warning signs are dyspnea, rales/crackles, and peripheral edema) or cardiac infarction.

Drug Interactions

- Beta blockers add to drug effects and can mask the onset of a hypoglycemic episode (e.g., tachycardia).
- Drugs interact with some diuretics like thiazide and loop diuretics, corticosteroids, and calcium channel blockers, which increase blood glucose levels. Risk of lactic acidosis with metformin is increased by a number of drugs including alcohol, morphine, calcium channel blockers, and ranitidine. Cross-sensitivity with sulfonamides occurs mostly with the sulfonylureas. Antifungal agents may interfere with glucose control of meglitinides.
- Glucosamine, chromium, and coenzyme Q10 may interfere with blood sugar control by hypoglycemic drugs.

Implications for Physical Therapists

- Make sure that the patient wears an identification tag or any other visible marker indicating that he or she is a diabetic. Also, make sure—depending on the drug—that the patient carries some sugar, a glucose preparation, or sweetened orange juice to counteract a hypoglycemic reaction.
- Do not recommend glucosamine to diabetic patients to treat joint problems unless this has been cleared with a physician, because glucosamine can cause hypoglycemic episodes in unadjusted hypoglycemic drug dosages.
- Be aware of the occurrence of hypoglycemia as well as hyperglycemia (unusual thirst, drowsiness, fruit-like breath, flushed). Treat the first with sugar (artificial sweeteners do not work) and the other by asking the patient to administer the needed drug dose.
- If you feel that a patient's blood glucose levels are fluctuating, ask if he or she has changed dietary habits or is using an OTC drug,

because these can be causes for poor glucose control.

- Exercise a diabetic patient, especially at the beginning of drug therapy carefully, because exercise can reduce blood glucose levels. Check glucose levels during and after exercise.

- If your patient is usually on metformin and complains about chills, dizziness, hypotension, muscle pain, bradycardia, and dyspnea, notify a physician immediately because these could be warning signs of ketoacidosis.

Immunomodulators

Common Drugs (selection of some of the most commonly used drugs)

Immunoinhibitors
DNA inhibitors
    Azathioprine (Azasan, Imuran)
    Cyclophosphamide (Cytoxan)
    Methotrexate (Trexal,
        Rheumatrex)
T-cell inactivators
    Cyclosporine (Neoral,
        Sandimmune, other)
    Sirolimus (Rapamune)
    Tacrolimus (Prograf, Protopic)
Gold compounds
    Auranofin (Ridaura)
    Other
NSAIDS (see NSAIDS)
Corticosteroids (see
    Corticosteroids)
Miscellaneous drugs
    Chloroquine (Aralen)
    Etanercept (Enbrel)
    Other
Immunostimulators
    Immunoglobulins Gamma
        globulin, Iveegam, Carimune,
        other
    Filgrastim (Neupogen)
    Sargramostim Leukine
    Other

Indications

Immunomodulators are indicated in:

- *Transplantation of tissues and organs*, in which the immune system tries to destroy foreign cells as it is supposed to do, but which in these cases is unwanted. Drugs like T cell inactivators reduce the activity of T cells, which are mostly involved in rejection reactions and this preserves the transplant.

- *Autoimmune diseases* such as rheumatoid arthritis, lupus erythematosus, polymyositis, myasthenia gravis, and others, where an exaggerated immune response damages healthy tissue and causes health problems. Drugs such as DNA inhibitors and gold compounds reduce the formation of immune cells (see both Antineoplastics and Corticosteroids) and reduce unwanted and excessive inflammations, reducing this response and preventing further damage. Chloroquine might act by damaging immune cells by changing their pH, and etanercept by blocking the action of the tumor necrosis factor.

- Other uses include stimulatory agents to increase white blood cell count during cancer chemotherapy. Filgrastim and sargramostim stimulate the formation of white blood cells in bone marrow.

Examples of Common Dosages
(general guidelines, many different dosage schedules)

Azathioprine: 1–3 mg/kg/day PO or 3–5 mg/kg IV

Cyclophosphamide: 1–2.5 mg/kg/day PO

Methotrexate: 7.5 mg/wk up to 20 mg/wk PO

Cyclosporine: 2.5–10 mg/kg/day once or divided doses PO

Sirolimus: 2 mg/day up to 5 mg/day PO

Tacrolimus: 0.03–0.05 mg/kg/day IV then 0.15 mg/kg 2 times daily PO

Auranofin: 6 mg once or 3 mg 2 times daily up to 9 mg/day PO

Chloroquine: 250 mg/day PO

Etanercept: 50 mg/wk SC

Filgrastim: 5–10 mcg/kg/day once IV SC INF

Sargramostim: 250–500 mcg/m2/day IV INF

Immunoglobulins: Various schedules

Administration

Most drugs are given PO but can be injected or used topically. Drugs are often administered in combination. In some cases, the response is delayed by weeks or months.

Contraindications

These drugs should not be used or must be used with caution in patients with immune system and blood problems.

Common Adverse Reactions

An adverse reaction to all immune suppressants is an increased risk of infections. Other adverse reactions differ among the groups (see also Antineoplastics, Anticancer drugs, NSAIDs, and Corticosteroids). T-cell inactivators can cause hepatic and renal damage, blood disorders, lung problems, seizures, and confusion. Gold compounds cause some GI distress but also some blood disorders such as leucopenia. Chloroquine is usually well-tolerated but might cause some retinal damage. Etanercept is more toxic and can cause serious infections, malignancies, and death.

Drug Interactions

- These drugs, depending on the class, can interact with a large number of other drugs.
- Ginseng and St. John's wort can decrease effectiveness of T-cell inactivators, and grapefruit juice can affect their bioavailability.

Implications for Physical Therapists

- Inform the patient about the difference between rheumatoid arthritis and osteoarthritis (the latter is somewhat of a misnomer because no inflammation is part of the causative process). Explain the use of NSAIDs that can be used in both conditions, whereas acetaminophen, which lacks antiinflammatory properties, can only be used in the latter situation.

- Inform the patient that foods rich in meat and proteins have been shown to aggravate, and foods high in fish oils to ameliorate, the signs of rheumatoid arthritis. Stress the importance of weight loss in overweight individuals because excessive weight worsens both conditions.
- Do not treat the patient, or be sure to wear a mask, if you have an infection (flu, respiratory infection, other) because immune suppressants increase the risk of an infection in these patients.
- Emphasize that muscle- and bone-strengthening exercise can be helpful in preventing further deterioration, particularly if corticosteroids are used.
- Observe the patient; if skin rashes or unexplained joint pain is experienced by the patient, this could indicate a more serious condition and might necessitate a change in drug.

Local Anesthetics

Common Drugs (selection of some of the most commonly used drugs)

Benzocaine (Anbesol, Lanacane, other [OTC])
Bupivacaine (Marcaine, Sensorcaine)
Dibucaine (Nupercainal)
Levobupivacaine (Chirocaine)
Lidocaine (Xylocaine, Dilocaine, other)
Procaine (Novocain)
Ropivacaine (Naropin)
Tetracaine (Pontocaine)

Indications

Local anesthetics are indicated in:

- *Surgery*, where blockade of pain impulses allows for analgesia during the surgical procedure. Drugs attach to sodium channels and do not allow the influx of sodium into the nerve. No action potential can occur, so pain impulses stop at this site and do not reach the brain. No pain can now be perceived and experienced.
- *Hypertonic muscles* (cerebrovascular accidents, head trauma) or *minor surface inflammation/irritation* (abrasions, burns). Drugs reduce or abolish pain sensation and decrease excessive feedback on efferent motor pathways.
- *Therapy of painful subcutaneous structures* (bursae, tendons) or *low back pain*. Drugs are applied topically with iontophoresis or phonophoresis, or in the last case, by patch. Again, pain sensation and muscle relaxation are achieved by blockade of nerve impulses.
- *Muscle spasms* where a "vicious" cycle keeps the muscle contracted. Drugs injected into the affected area break this cycle by interfering with nerve impulses, and thus relax the muscle.

Examples of Common Dosages
(general guidelines, many different dosage schedules)

Benzocaine: Various preparations

Bupivacaine: 25–100 mg as a 0.5% solution epidural

Dibucaine: Various preparations

Levobupivacaine: 50–150 mg as a 0.5% solution epidural

Lidocaine: 300 mg IM or 50–100 mg IV

Procaine: 50–100 mg for spinal anesthesia

Ropivacaine: 12–16 mg epidural

Tetracaine: Various routes and dosages

Administration

These drugs, such as benzocaine, dibucaine, and tetracaine, are used topically, either alone or assisted by iontophoresis or phonophoresis, or by injection or infiltration. Some drugs are applied as patches. In some cases, alpha agonists are added to injectable preparations to cause vasoconstriction, which allows smaller amounts of the local anesthetic to remain for a longer time at the injection site.

Contraindications

These drugs should not be used or must be used with caution in patients with cardiac and hepatic diseases. This applies mostly to injections.

Common Adverse Reactions

Adverse reactions differ among drugs. In general, no major toxicities are expected with topical appli-cation unless very large doses are used. In the case of injections, car-diotoxicity (bradycardia, dysrhyth-mias, and hypotension) and CNS effects (tinnitus, agitation, restless-ness, confusion, tremors, twitching, dizziness, fainting, and seizures) can be expected. Repeated injec-tions into the same place can cause muscle pain and necrosis.

Drug Interactions

Interactions occur mostly after injections with other drugs.

Implications for Physical Therapists

- Drugs allow the physical thera-pist to do manipulations and rehabilitation techniques without inflicting unnecessary pain.
- Patients with infiltration therapy might experience hypotension, sensory impairments and motor deficits. Patients must be watched carefully when walking and when getting up to avoid falls. As a pre-caution, these functions should be tested before therapy.
- Patients with infiltration therapy might have abolished or de-creased pain perception, and thermal and electrical stimuli must be applied with care. As a precaution, sensory functions should be tested before therapy.
- Watch out for tinnitus, agita-tion, tremors, and confusion in patients with epidural therapy, because this could indicate an overdose reaction requiring dosage adjustments.

Male Hormones

Common Drugs (selection of some of the most commonly used drugs)

Androgens
  Testosterone (Andronate, Dura-test, other)
  Nandrolone (Hybolin, Kabolin)
  Other
Antiandrogens
  Finasteride (Proscar)
  Dutasteride (Avodart)
  Other

Indications

Male hormones are indicated in:

- *Replacement therapy* when there is a deficiency state, such as after removal of testes, hypogonadism, and other forms of under-functiong testosterone. Testosterone or its analogues are administered to fulfill the function of a deficiency or lack of the endogenous hormone.
- *Benign prostatic hyperplasia*, in which the prostate is enlarged and interferes with normal urination. Antidrogens inhibit the conversion of testerone to the more active dihydrotesterone, which promotes prostate growth and actually shrinks an enlarged prostate, reducing urinary problems.
- Other uses include certain *anemias*.

Examples of Common Dosages

(general guidelines, many different dosage schedules)

Testosterone: 25–50 mg 2–3 times a week or 100 mg/month IM
Nandrolone: 100–200 mg/week IM
Finasteride: 5 mg/day PO
Dutasteride: 0.5 mg/day PO

Administration

Depending on the drug, they are given PO, IM, or by patch.

Contraindications

These drugs should not be used or must be used with caution in patients with renal/cardiac and/or hepatic disease.

Common Adverse Reactions

- Adverse reactions differ, but androgens may affect blood glucose levels and may cause jaundice. Antiandrogens decrease libido and sexual performance.
- In cases of abuse of very high doses of androgens, over long periods of time by athletes trying to increase bone and muscle mass as well as performance (although it is still uncertain how much these androgens actually contribute to increased muscle mass and performance), number and intensity of adverse reactions increase markedly. Abuse has been associated with liver problems that can be fatal; cardiomyopathy; and other heart diseases, dysrhythmias, and bone damage.

Drug Interactions

These drugs can interact with a number of drugs.

Implications for Physical Therapists

If an athletic person with well-developed muscles is seen, inquire about illegal use of androgens. Inform this individual that these substances might not do what he or she expects them to do, but that they can significantly increase the risk of adverse reactions. These can signifi- cantly shorten life expectancy—in other words, they can cause an early death. Athletes often trust physical therapists more than other health professionals.

Miscellaneous Vasodilators

Common Drugs (selection of some of the most commonly used drugs)

Peripherally acting vasodilators
   Hydralazine (Apresoline)
   Other
Centrally acting vasodilators
   Clonidine (Catapres)
   Other
Vasodilators for erectile
   dysfunction
   Sildenafil (Viagra)
   Vardenafil (Levitra)
   Tadalafil (Cialis)
   Other
Antianginals
   Isosorbide (Dilatrate, Isordil,
     other)
   Nitroglycerin (Nitrocot,
     Nitro-Time, Nitrogard,
     other)

Indications

These drugs are indicated in:

- *Hypertension*, when increased cardiac output and/or peripheral resistance increases blood pressure. Hypertension left untreated is linked to myocardial infarctions and strokes. Vasodilators such as hydralazine, which increases the vasodilating metabolite c-GMP and clonidine, which reduces central sympathetic outflow, dilate blood ves- sels and reduce blood pressure, and can reduce the risk of sec- ondary myocardial infarctions and strokes.

- *Angina*, where insufficient blood flow (e.g., atherosclerosis) does not supply enough oxygen to cardiac muscle. Under emotional or physical stress, heart rate and contractility increase, causing them to exceed the oxygen supply and cause anginal pain. Antiangi- nals, which form NO and c-GMP, dilate coronary blood vessels, which increases cardiac blood flow and oxygen supply to the heart.

- *Erectile dysfunction* is an inability to initiate and/or maintain an erection. An erection begins with sensory or mental stimulation, allowing the muscles of the corpora cavernosa to relax and the penis to fill with blood. This relaxation is initiated and main- tained by cGMP. Drugs increase and maintain levels of c-GMP by blocking its destruction by the special phosphodiesterase or PDE5.

- *Opioid withdrawal and pain man- agement* in cancer patients who don't respond to opioids might involve the use of clonidine.

Examples of Common Dosages

(general guidelines, many different dosage schedules)

Hydralazine: 10–50 mg 4 times daily (not to exceed 320 mg/day) PO

Clonidine: 0.1–0.6 mg 2 times daily PO

Sildenafil: 25–100 mg taken 30–60 min before sexual activity PO

Vardenafil: 5–20 mg taken 60 min before sexual activity PO

Tadalafil: 5–20 mg 15 min prior to sexual activity PO

Isosorbide: 2.5–10 mg every 5–10 min for 3 doses sl or 5–40 mg every 6 hrs PO (Dinitrate)

Nitroglycerin: 0.3–0.6 mg every 5 min for 15 min sl or 1 mg every 5 hours buccal; 2.5–9 mg every 8 hr for extended release capsules or 0.1–0.6 mg/hr by patch

Administration

These drugs are given PO or by injections usually only in hospitals. Clonidine can be given by transdermal or epidural administration. Antianginals can be given sublingually. Vasodilators for erectile dysfunction have a similar onset (between 30 to 60 minutes) but last between 4 to 36 hours (tadalafil). Antianginals have a very quick (few minutes) onset of action and are used to prevent or abort an attack of angina.

Contraindications

These drugs are contraindicated in cases of hypersensitivity. Drugs should be used with caution in cases of renal or hepatic impairments. Vasodilators for erectile dysfunction should not be used in individuals with cardiovascular disease for 6 months after a myocardial infarction.

Common Adverse Reactions

Peripheral vasodilators can cause tachycardia, hypotension, sodium retention (edema), and a syndrome resembling lupus. Central vasodilators can cause drowsiness, dry mouth, and bradycardia, and should not be discontinued abruptly. Vasodilators for erectile dysfunction can cause headache, nasal decongestion, vision loss (rare), GI problems, flushing, cardiovascular collapse, and priapism (erection lasting longer than 4 hours). Antianginals may cause hypotension, tachycardia, dizziness, and headaches.

Drug Interactions

Peripheral vasodilators can increase the antihypertensive effects of other antihypertensives and alcohol. Central vasodilators increase sedative effects of drugs with similar effects. Vasodilators for erectile dysfunction should not be used with antihypertensive drugs, in particular with alcohol, nitrates, or alpha antagonists because of the possibility of severe hypotension. Antianginals should be used with caution with beta blockers, and not at all with vasodilators used for erectile dysfunction.

Implications for Physical Therapists

- Advise patients to change positions and get up slowly,

because orthostatic hypotension may occur. This is mostly in the beginning of therapy and in geriatric individuals.

- If patients complain about unexplained joint pain, notify or have patients contact their physician, as this could be a lupus-like syndrome.
- If you notice peripheral edemas such as swollen ankles, notify or have patients contact their physician, as this could be caused by excessive sodium retention.

- Be aware that central vasodilators may cause drowsiness, which can interfere with the physical therapy routine. This should slowly diminish during therapy.
- If the patient has an attack of angina and responds to nitroglycerin, have them get up slowly because orthostatic hypotension might occur. If the patient does not respond to 3 doses of nitroglycerin, call 911 because this could signal a myocardial infarction.

Nonnarcotic Analgesics

Common Drugs (selection of some of the most commonly used drugs)

Acetaminophen (Tylenol, Abenol, Aceta, Dapacin, Dynafed, other [OTC])

Diclofenac (Cataflam, Voltaren, Solaraze)

Etodolac (Lodine)

Ibuprofen (Motrin, Advil, Nuprin, Actiprofen, Genpril [OTC])

Ketoprofen (Actron, Orudis, Oruvail, Rhodis, Apo-Keto)

Ketorolac (Toradol)

Meloxicam (Mobic)

Naproxen (Aleve, Anaprox, Naprosyn, Synflex, Naprelan, other [OTC])

Salicylates (acetyl-) (Aspirin, Acuprin, Arthrisin, other [aspirin is acetylsalicylic acid to be metabolized to active metabolite salicylic acid {OTC}])

Salicylates, (Tricosal, Anaflex, Arthropan, other)

Other
(See also Nonsteroidal Antiinflammatory Drugs [NSAIDs])

Indications

Drugs are indicated in:

- *Mild to moderate* pain caused by trauma, headaches, toothaches, muscle soreness and aches, dysmenorrhea, osteoarthritis, and inflammatory disorders such as rheumatoid arthritis and bursitis. Drugs inhibit the enzyme cyclooxygenase (COX-I and COX-II) and reduce or prevent synthesis of prostaglandins. These initiate (with other compounds) impulse formation in pain fibers. Drugs show similar analgesic actions with some exceptions. Ketorolac has been found to be particularly effective for postoperative pain. Drugs are most effective if taken early on, at the onset of pain.

Some patients will show a better response to one drug but not another. Higher doses than those recommended usually do not provide for more pain relief. Dosages for analgesic effects are usually lower than those for inflammatory conditions.

- *Prevention of blood clot formation*, where aspirin in small doses (e.g., 81 mg) has been shown to reduce thrombi formation, which is one of the causative factors in heart attacks and strokes. Aspirin reduces formation of prostaglandins and the related thromboxane, which are involved in platelet aggregation. Other drugs have less of an antiplatelet effect, and acetaminophen has none.

Examples of Common Dosages
(general guidelines, many different dosage schedules)

Acetaminophen: 650–1000 mg every 4–6 hrs (up to 4 g per day) PO

Aspirin: 325–500 mg every 4 hrs (not to exceed 4 g) PO

Diclofenac: 100 mg initially and / or 25–50 mg every 6 hrs PO

Etodolac: 200–400 mg every 6 hrs (not to exceed 1200 mg) PO

Ibuprofen: 200–400 mg every 5 hrs (not to exceed 1200 mg) PO

Ketoprofen: 25–50 mg every 6 hrs (not to exceed 75 mg) PO

Ketorolac: 20 mg followed by 10 mg every 5 hrs (not to exceed 20 doses/days and not more than 5 days) PO

Meloxicam: 7.5 mg once a day PO

Naproxen: 250–400 mg and 250 mg every 6 hrs (not to exceed 1.5 g). Slow-release preparation 375–500 mg 2 times a day PO

Administration
These drugs are used mostly orally. They are best taken with a large glass of water or food while staying in an upright position for about 30 minutes. Onset of action is usually 15 to 30 minutes. Duration of action varies among drugs but is generally between 4 and 8 hours (slow-release preparations can increase duration).

Contraindications
Contraindications to the use of these drugs include hypersensitivity, GI problems (gastritis, ulcer), and renal and hepatic disorders.

Common Adverse Reactions
- All drugs can cause abdominal pain, dyspepsia, and GI bleeding (tarry stools are indicative of internal bleeding). Some drugs can be photosensitizing. Hypersensitivity reactions are rare, and they occur more frequently if the patients are sensitive to aspirin and have asthma and nasal polyps (except with acetaminophen). Drugs can be toxic to the liver and show renal toxicity, but mostly in individuals with already compromised hepatic and renal functions. They can slightly increase the risk of cardiovascular events, again mostly during chronic use and in individuals with cardiovascular problems.

- Acetaminophen causes fewer GI problems but is more liver toxic and can affect blood glucose monitoring. Ketoprofen has a higher incidence of headache and dizziness. Aspirin should not be used in children with viral infections because it can cause the potentially fatal Reye syndrome (acetaminophen is the drug of choice in these cases).

Drug Interactions

There is an increased risk of GI problems (gastritis, ulcer) enhanced by concurrent use of spicy foods, alcohol, and some herbal products such as arnica, garlic, and ginseng. Acetaminophen plus alcohol (more than two glasses of wine or beer) has been associated with increased liver toxicity.

Implications for Physical Therapists

- Patients often report only prescription drugs when asked about drug use. Because some analgesics are also obtained without a prescription, the question should also include use of OTC drugs (and vitamins/herbal medications). Advise patients that OTC drugs must be used with caution.
- Analgesics may mask pain during mobility movements. This can lead to damage by exceeding movement limitations or by providing the impression of mobility that is not as good as imagined.
- Extensive UV radiation should be avoided or body parts should be covered because some drugs can cause photosensitivity reactions.
- Some patients may experience drowsiness and might exhibit slight incoordination, but this is very rare with these drugs.
- Advise patients to use acetaminophen for low back pain, because a recent study suggests that this drug seems to be most effective and carries the fewest side effects.
- Advise patients that OTC analgesics should not be taken for longer than 2 weeks without consulting a physician, because they can mask a serious underlying health problem.

Nonsteroidal Antiinflammatory Drugs or NSAIDs

Common Drugs (selection of some of the most commonly used drugs)

Diclofenac (Cataflam, Voltaren, Solaraze)

Etodolac (Lodine)

Ibuprofen (Motrin, Advil, Nuprin, Actiprofen, Genpril [OTC available])

Indomethacin (Indocin, Indocron, other)

Ketoprofen (Actron, Orudis, Oruvail, Rhodis, Apo-Keto)

Ketorolac (Toradol)

Meloxicam (Mobic)

Nabumetone (Relafen)

Naproxen (Aleve, Anaprox, Naprosyn, Synflex, Naprelan, other [OTC available])

Oxaprozin (Daypro)

Piroxicam (Feldene)

Sulindac (Clinoril)

Salicylates (acetyl-) Aspirin, Acuprin, Arthrisin, other (composed of acetylsalicylic acid to be metabolized to active metabolite salicylic acid (OTC available)

Salicylates, (Tricosal, Anaflex, Arthropan, other)

Tolmetin (Tolectin)

Celecoxib (Celebrex)

(See also Nonnarcotic Analgesics and Corticosteroids)

Indications

NSAIDS are indicated in:

- *Inflammations*, which are characterized by swelling, redness, warmth and pain, and eventual tissue damage if they become excessive, as in certain autoimmune diseases, transplants, allergies, asthma, croup, rheumatoid arthritis, osteoarthritis, ankylosing spondylitis, bursitis, and other conditions. Drugs curtail excessive and reduce unwanted inflammations to protect healthy tissue. Drugs inhibit cyclooxygenase (COX I and II) and reduce or prevent synthesis of prostaglandins, which initiate and maintain inflammatory processes by vasodilatation. Drugs often work best when taken at the beginning of an inflammatory process. Indomethacin is one of the strongest antiinflammatory drugs but also carries the more severe adverse reactions.

- *Dysmenorrhea*, in which excessive prostaglandin formation stimulates the uterus, causing painful contractions. Drugs reduce prostaglandin levels, excessive contractions, and cramps.

- *Fever*, which is initiated by a central action of prostaglandins on the area which regulates body temperature. Drugs reduce prostaglandin formation and lower fever.

- *Actinic keratosis* (diclofenac) and *ocular inflammations* after surgery; *allergic conjunctivitis* and *inhibition of perioperative miosis* (bromfenac, diclofenac, flurbipro-fen, ketorolac, nepafenac, suprofen).

Examples of Common Dosages
(general guidelines, many different dosage schedules)

Acetaminophen: 650–1000 mg every 4–6 hrs (up to 4 g per day) PO

Aspirin: 325–500 mg every 4 hrs (not to exceed 4 g) PO

Diclofenac: 50–100 mg 3–4 times daily PO

Etodolac: 300 mg 2–3 times daily or 400–1200 mg once daily as extended release preparation PO

Ibuprofen: 400–800 mg 3–4 times daily (not to exceed 3600 mg/ day) PO

Indomethacin: 25–50 mg 2–4 times daily or 75 mg once daily with extended release preparations PO

Ketoprofen: 150–300 mg/day in 3–4 divided dose or 100–200 mg once daily with extended release preparations PO

Ketorolac: 20 mg followed by 10 mg every 5 hrs (not to exceed 40 mg/day) PO

Meloxicam: 7.5–15 mg once a day PO

Naproxen: 250–500 mg 2–3 times a day (not to exceed 1.5 g) or 375–500 mg twice a day with the slow release preparation PO

Nabumetone: 1000–2000 mg once or twice a day PO

Oxaprozin: 1200–1800 mg once daily PO

Piroxicam: 10–20 mg once or twice a day PO

Sulindac: 150–200 mg twice a day PO

Tolmetin: 400–1800 mg/day in 3 divided dose (not to exceed 2000 mg/day) PO

Celecoxib: 100–200 mg once or twice a day PO

Administration

These drugs can be given IV or PO. They are best taken with meals or a large glass of water while sitting up/standing for 30 minutes after ingestion of the drug.

Contraindications

Contraindications include hypersensitivity to a drug, which often manifests itself as hypersensitivity to the entire group, and GI problems (gastritis, ulcers). They should be used cautiously in cases of severe hepatic, renal, and cardiovascular diseases.

Common Adverse Reactions

Adverse reactions include dizziness, drowsiness, abdominal distress, dyspepsia, gastritis, ulcer, photosensitivity, and after long-term use, nephritis. Rarely, they can cause Stevens-Johnson syndrome, hepatitis, or exfoliate dermatitis. Celecoxib is a COX II inhibitor and somewhat gentler on the stomach but can increase the risk of cardiovascular accidents. Patients with nasal polyps, asthma, or aspirin-induced allergy are at high risk to develop hypersensitivity reactions towards other drugs.

Drug Interactions

- They can interact with a large number of drugs, such as enhancing the effects of warfarin and related drugs, increasing bleeding times; or decreasing the effects of antihypertensives and insulin. Alcohol increases adverse effects on the stomach.
- Arnica, dong quai, garlic, ginseng, and ginkgo increase the risk of bleeding. Spicy foods aggravate stomach problems.

Implications for Physical Therapists

- Patients often report only prescription drugs when asked about drug use. Because some NSAIDs are also obtained without a prescription, the question should also include use of prescription as well as OTC drugs (and vitamins/herbal medications).
- Advise patients that antiinflammatory OTC drugs are drugs and must be used with caution, and patients must adhere to the warning statements on the container.
- NSAIDs may mask pain during mobility movements and can give the impression of better mobility than actually exists. This can cause damage if patients exceed movement limitations.

- Extensive UV radiation should be avoided or body parts should be covered because some drugs cause photosensitization.
- Some patients may experience drowsiness and might exhibit slight incoordination, but this is very rare with these drugs.
- If patients complain about stomach problems, tell them to take medications with a lot of water or a meal while sitting up or standing for at least 30 minutes afterward. Patients should also watch their stool, and if black (occult bleeding), should stop the drug and notify a physician immediately.
- If patients complain about an upper respiratory infection, cough, muscle aching, and a rash with blisters, ask them to contact a physician immediately, because this could be a sign of Stevens-Johnson syndrome.
- If you notice dry, itchy, red areas on hands and other parts of the body, have patients notify a physician immediately, because this could be exfoliate dermatitis.
- Explain to patients that acetaminophen is not antiinflammatory and should not be used if an antiinflammatory drug has been prescribed.

Opioid or Narcotic Analgesics

Common Drugs (selection of some of the most commonly used drugs)

Butorphanol (Stadol)
Buprenorphine (Buprenex, Subutex)
Codeine (Paveral)
Fentanyl (Actiq, Sublimaze, Duragesic [transdermal])
Hydrocodone (Hycodan, Robidone)
   In combination with acetaminophen (Anexsia, Bancap, Dolacet, other)
   In combination with aspirin (Alor, Azdone, other)
   In combination with ibuprofen (Vicoprofen)
Hydromorphone (Dilaudid, Hydrostat)
Meperidine (Demerol, Pethidine)

Methadone (Dolophine, Methadose)
Morphine (Astramorph, Avinza, Epimorph, Roxanol, other)
Nalbuphine (Nubain)
Oxycodone (Endocodone, OxyContin, Percolone, Roxicodone)
Oxymorphone (Numorphan)
Pentazocine (Talwin
   In combination with acetaminophen (Talacen)
   In combination with aspirin (Talwin compound)
Propoxyphene (Darvon)
   In combination with aspirin (Darvon-N c ASA)
   In combination with aspirin and caffeine (Darvon 32 or 65)
   In combination with acetaminophen (Darvocet)

Indications

Opioid or narcotic analgesics are indicated in:

- *Moderate to severe pain* of all kinds, which is often measured on a subjective scale of 0 to 10. Drugs stimulate opioid receptors μ, κ, δ in the CNS, which are physiologically activated by endogenous compounds such as enkephalins, endorphins, and dynorphines, and which prevent pain impulses from reaching their central destination. Activation of these receptors causes analgesia and pain is reduced, felt less, or is completely gone. Drugs work best for analgesia if given at the onset of pain. The patient is usually the best person to asses and request the medication and not a pre-prescribed schedule (although overdoses must be avoided).
- *Therapy of opioid dependence and withdrawal* (buprenorphine, methadone), *cough* (codeine, hydrocodone, hydromorphone), *diarrhea* (codeine), and before and during *surgery* (fentanyl, meperidine, nalbuphine). Drugs act on opioid receptors and reduce withdrawal, cough, and diarrhea.

Examples of Common Dosages

(general guidelines, many different dosage schedules)

Butorphanol: 1–2 mg q 3–4 hr IM, IV; 1 mg as nasal spray q 3–4 hr

Buprenorphine: 0.3 mg q 4–6 hr IM, IV

Morphine: 10–30 mg q 3–4 hr PO; 4–15 mg q 3–4 hr IM

Pentazocine: 50–100 mg q 3–4 hrs PO (up to 600 mg/day); 30 mg q 3–4 hr IM, IV
  (plus acetaminophen: 25 mg and 650 mg)
  (plus aspirin: 12.5 mg and 325 mg)

Codeine: 15–60 mg q 3–6 hr PO; 15–60 mg q 4–6 hr IM, IV
  (plus acetaminophen: 30–60 mg and 300 mg)
  (plus aspirin: 60 mg and 325 mg)

Fentanyl: 200 mcg dissolved in mouth (higher doses available up to 1600 mcg); 0,5–1 mcg/kg to be repeated every 60 min IV

Hydrocodone: 2.5–10 mg q 3–6 hr PO
  (plus acetaminophen: 5 mg and 500 mg)
  (plus aspirin: 5 mg and 500 mg)
  (plus ibuprofen: 7.5 mg and 200 mg)

Hydromorphone: 4–8 mg q 3–4 hr PO; 1.5 mg q 3–4 hr IM, IV, SC

Meperidine: 50–150 mg q 3–4 hr PO, IM, IV (short-term use only)

Methadone: 20 mg q 7 hr PO; 10 mg q 7 hr IM, SC

Nalbuphine: 10 mg q 3–6 hr (total dose 160 mg) IV, IM

Oxycodone: 5–10 mg q 3–4 hr PO

Oxymorphone: 0.5 mg q 3–6 hr IV; 1–1.5 mg q 3–6 hr SC, IM

Propoxyphene: 65 mg q 4 hr (not to exceed 390 mg) PO
  (plus aspirin: 100 mg and 325 mg)
  (plus aspirin and caffeine: 32 mg or 65 mg, 389 mg, 30 mg)
  (plus acetaminophen: 50, 65, or 100 mg, 325, 500, or 650 mg)

(See also Nonnarcotic Analgesics)

Administration

Drugs can be given orally, rectally, IM, IV, by infusion pump ("patient-controlled analgesia"), or patch (fentanyl). Onset of action after oral use is about 30 minutes, and duration of action varies but can be increased with sustained release tablets. Injections provide relief in minutes.

Contraindications

Contraindications to the use of these drugs include hypersensitivity, head trauma, and increased intracranial pressure.

Common Adverse Reactions

All drugs cause sedation, drowsiness, incoordination, and some respiratory depression (in particular in geriatric patients). Most patients suffer from constipation (which might require the use of laxatives). Some individuals experience nausea and vomiting, which can be avoided by assuming a supine position, and hypotension, which is more marked when quickly assuming an upright position. Miosis interferes with vision in dim or dark conditions. Chronic use of these drugs can lead to physical dependence and tolerance (except miosis and constipation, which do not show tolerance). In case of tolerance, changing to another drug is often beneficial. Some drugs are prone to be abused including heroin, which is converted to morphine in the body.

Drug Interactions

These drugs should not be used in patients receiving MAO inhibitors for depression. There is an increased risk of sedation and CNS depression with drugs that also cause CNS depression, as well as alcohol, valerian, chamomile, and kava.

Implications for Physical Therapists

- Analgesics may make movement exercises easier by reducing pain. They also may mask pain during mobility movements and can cause damage if patients exceed movement limitations. Drugs might feign or give the impression of better mobility than actually exists.
- If manipulations under opioid analgesia must be made that would otherwise be painful, arrange therapy at the peak of the drug's effects, usually 2 hours after use of the drug.
- Assess alertness of patients because they can be more or less sedated, drowsy, and uncoordinated, and certain tasks requiring attention and quick reflexes should be modified or omitted.
- Ask patients to change positions slowly, particularly from a lying to a standing position, to avoid orthostatic hypotension. Orthostatic hypotension can cause the patient to become dizzy, and faint and fall.
- Respiration depression must be considered when using exercise because reducing the exercise-induced respiratory rate can lead to hypoxia.
- If patients have to lie on their backs for longer periods and breathe very shallowly, ask patients to take a few deep breaths every 30 minutes to expand their

lungs (to reduce risk of lung collapse).
- During withdrawal from chronic use of one of these drugs, diffuse muscle discomfort might occur, This can be alleviated with heat or massages.

OTC Drugs

Introduction

Over-the-counter (OTC) drugs are nonprescription medications that can be obtained without a prescription. Classification as an OTC drug is based on three criteria: 1) The consumer must be able to easily understand the medical condition to be treated and monitor its progress; 2) the drug must have a favorable adverse reaction profile; and 3) drug administration must be simple and easy.

Although these drugs are indeed efficacious and have a low adverse reaction profile, they nevertheless can show adverse reactions, mask serious medical problems, be used for the wrong reasons, be used incorrectly, and interact with prescription drugs.

Consumers must carefully read labels to avoid further medical problems. For example, consumers must be aware of the medical condition, of how much and for how long to use the medication, of other medical conditions that might preclude using this drug, and of which prescription drugs or other substances might interact with the medication. OTC drugs must always be mentioned to a physician. Consumers must be aware that some ingredients are not obvious, such as ethanol or caffeine, which can cause their own effects. Also, OTC drugs should not be used when pregnant or breast-feeding unless advised by a physician, because some drugs can reach the fetus or infant through the placenta or milk.

Consumers should not give adult drugs to infants or small children, unless it is stated on the label that it is okay to do so. also, many infant and children preparations recently had to be removed from the market after they were found to be either not necessary or toxic to infants.

Consumers must be observant when treating a problem. If two tablets are recommended, but a person is small or older, then it is advisable to start with one tablet. Only if there is no relief should the dose be increased. Similarly, an obese person might need three tablets instead of the recommended two.

Major adverse reactions to watch out for include:

Analgesics: GI discomfort, rebound headaches, bleeding, interactions with antiinflammatory drugs and anticoagulants

Acetaminophen: liver damage with moderate to high doses of ethanol; also note that acetaminophen is analgesic and antipyretic but not antiinflammatory

Antihistamines: drowsiness, urinary hesitancy/retention (in the elderly), contact lens intolerance, enhanced sedation with alcohol (has been used in date-rape cases)

Decongestants: increased blood pressure, counteraction of antihypertensive medications, rebound effect with prolonged use of nasal preparations

H2 blockers: dysrhythmias, constipation, agranulocytosis

Pump inhibitors: liver and renal problems, neutropenia

Vaginal creams: headache, missed menstrual periods, fever

Emergency contraceptives (Plan B—postcoital pill): nausea, vomiting, stomach pain, dizziness, headache, diarrhea

Implications for Physical Therapists

- The physical therapist can play an important role in advising patients on the use of OTC drugs or in suggesting the use of such drugs, because many patients might not read the entire label or might not understand its use or content.

- Patients must be advised that OTC medications are drugs that can produce serious adverse reactions if used improperly, and that their physicians must be contacted if these occur.

- All OTC medications must be mentioned in a medical history to avoid detrimental interactions with prescription drugs.

- Advise patients about the difference between antiinflammatory drugs and acetaminophen, which is not antiinflammatory.

- Advise patients that use of acetaminophen with even moderate doses of alcohol can damage the liver.

- Advise patients that topical drugs will be absorbed into the body and that use of excessive amounts can cause serious systemic effects.

- Physical therapists can warn individuals with rebound headaches (no relief and even worse headaches in spite of drug use) that continued and excessive use of analgesics for headaches can exacerbate the problem. They can instead suggest relaxation techniques, massages, or gentle exercises.

Sedatives-Hypnotics

Common Drugs (selection of some of the most commonly used drugs)

Hypnotic benzodiazepines
    Flurazepam (Dalmane)
    Temazepam (Restoril, Razepam)
    Triazolam (Halcion)
Miscellaneous hypnotics
    Zaleplon (Sonata)

    Zolpidem (Ambien)
    Other
Barbiturates
    Secobarbital (Seconal)
    Pentobarbital (Nembutal)
    Other
OTC product
    Melatonin

Indications

Sedatives-hypnotics are mainly indicated in:

- *Insomnia*, which is a sleep disorder characterized by a persistent difficulty in falling asleep or staying asleep. It is usually followed by tiredness and functional impairment the next day.
- Hypnotic drugs—dose dependent—enhance GABA action, leading first to sedation and finally hypnosis. Barbiturates are generally more sleep inducing, whereas the others are more sleep promoting. Drugs that are quickly absorbed and have a short duration of action are helpful in the initiation of sleep (e.g., triazolam), whereas drugs with a slow rate of absorption and long duration of action keep individuals asleep longer (e.g., flurazepam).
- Other conditions like *epilepsy* (see *Anticonvulsants*), *movement disorders* (see *Skeletal Muscle Relaxants*), or anxiety (see *Anxiolytics*).

Examples of Common Dosages
(general guidelines, many different dosage schedules)

Flurazepam: 15–30 mg once PO
Temazepam: 7.5–30 mg PO
Triazolam: 0.125–0.5 mg PO
Zaleplon: 10–20 mg PO
Zolpidem: 10 mg (for 10 days only) PO
Pentobarbital: 100–200 mg PO
Secobarbital: 100–200 mg PO
Melatonin: 0.5–50 mg PO

Administration

These drugs are taken at bedtime orally. Barbiturates are sometimes injected or given rectally.

Contraindications

These drugs should not be used in (or must be used with caution in) patients with renal and hepatic diseases.

Common Adverse Reactions

Common adverse reactions are residual effects that might cause individuals to be drowsy, and have decreased motor function and muscular coordination the next day. This occurs mostly in older individuals. All drugs—to varying degrees—cause tolerance and physical dependence, so long-term treatment should not be discontinued abruptly. Withdrawal syndrome might manifest itself in irritation, excitation, and insomnia (and, rarely, convulsions). High doses can cause some respiratory depression. Other adverse reactions are usually mild. Some individuals might experience anterograde amnesia (forgetting events that took place before the drug was consumed). Zolpidem might cause "sleep eating."

Drug Interactions

The action of these drugs, in particular the residual effects, is enhanced in the presence of other drugs with sedative effects, including alcohol.

Sedative effects are increased by a number of herbs including chamomile, mistletoe, and valerian. St.

John's wort seems to reduce their effectiveness.

Implications for Physical Therapists

- If patients using these drugs appear drowsy and uncoordinated in morning sessions, schedule these patients in the afternoon when most aftereffects should have disappeared. Warn them not to drive if they feel drowsy.
- Warn patients not to discontinue drugs abruptly after long-term use by themselves but to first consult their physician. They might otherwise experience withdrawal symptoms.

- Tell patients not to drink or eat products containing caffeine because they can decrease drug effectiveness, and those products might even be a cause of the sleep problem.
- If a patient on zolpidem notices weight gain without having changed eating habits, ask the patient to notify the physician because the patient might be "sleep eating."
- The physical therapist can also suggest relaxation techniques, exercises, or massages to reduce the need for sleep medications.

Skeletal Muscle Relaxants

Common Drugs (selection of some of the most commonly used drugs)

Centrally acting drugs
 Baclofen (Lioresal)
 Carisoprodol (Soma, Vanadom)
 Chlorzoxazone (Paraflex, Parafon, other)
 Cyclobenzaprine (Flexeril, other)
 Diazepam (Valium, other)
 Gabapentin (Neurontin)
 Metaxalone (Skelaxin)
 Methocarbamol (Carbacot, Robaxin, other)
 Orphenadrine (Antiflex, Norflex)
 Tizanidine (Zanaflex)
Direct-acting drugs
 Dantrolene (Dantrium)
 Dichlorodifluoromethane

Neuromuscular-blocking drugs
 Botulinum toxin A (Botox)
 Botulinum toxin B (Myobloc)

Indications

Skeletal muscle relaxants are indicated in:

- *Spasticity*, which is characterized by excessive skeletal muscle excitation and contraction (exaggerated muscle stretch reflex). It is caused by central pathology as in multiple sclerosis, cerebral palsy, injury, or stroke, and it occurs when supraspinal control is lost. The drugs act by increasing the action of the inhibitory neurotransmitter GABA (diazepam, baclofen, gabapentin), blocking alpha receptors (tizanidine), or reducing excessive calcium fluxes in skeletal muscles (dantrolene).

- *Spasm*, which is characterized by increased muscle tension because of muscle injury, inflammation, and other causes. Frequently used drugs are carisoprodol, methocarbamol, cyclobenzaprine, and chlorzoxazone. Drugs seem to act in the spinal cord by suppressing polysynaptic reflex activity with uncertain mechanisms. Dichlorodifluoromethane cools the area and slows muscular and nervous activity. In severe cases (dystonia), botulinum toxin is injected, which destroys temporarily the terminals of the motor neurons and prevents the release of acetylcholine, causing actual muscle paralysis. After this time, new terminals are synthesized. Duration of action is up to 3 months.
- *Malignant hyperthermia, tetanus, seizures, neuralgia, and cosmetic purposes*: Botulinum injections to remove wrinkles.

Examples of Common Dosages
(general guidelines, many different dosage schedules)

Baclofen: 5–20 mg 3 times daily up to 80 mg/day PO

Carisoprodol: 350 mg 3 times daily PO

Chlorzoxazone: 250–750 mg 3–4 times daily PO

Cyclobenzaprine: 5 mg 3 times daily up to 30 mg/day PO

Diazepam: 2–10 mg 3–4 times daily or 15–30 mg extended release preparations PO

Gabapentin: 900–1800 mg/day in 3 divided doses PO

Metaxalone: 800 mg 3–4 times daily PO

Methocarbamol: 1–1.5 g 3–4 times daily PO

Orphenadrine: 100 mg 2 times daily PO

Tizanidine: 8 mg 3–4 times daily PO

Dantrolene: 25–100 mg 2–4 times daily PO

Dichlorodifluoromethane: Spray

Botulinum toxin A: 200–300 units IM, SC

Botulinum toxin B: 2500–5000 units IM, SC

Administration

Most drugs are given PO but can be injected or delivered by pumps (as with intrathecal baclofen). Drugs might be started at a low dose, which can be gradually increased. Botulinum toxin is only injected IM or SC. Dichlorodifluoromethane is applied topically as a spray.

Contraindications

These drugs should not be used in (or must be used with caution in) patients with hepatic diseases. Baclofen and dantrolene should not be used in patients who use spasticity to partially maintain balance.

Common Adverse Reactions

All drugs will cause sedation, drowsiness, and muscle weakness, as well as GI distress to a varying degree. Older individuals may experience periods of confusion. Some drugs might cause physical dependence and should not be discontinued abruptly. Drugs like baclofen, carisoprodol, and methocarbamol can precipitate seizures in patients, but mostly in those with a history of seizures. Chlorzoxazone has been associated with hepatitis, GI bleeding, and anemia.

Drug Interactions

- Sedation is increased with all drugs that also carry sedative properties, such as antihistamines, alcohol, antidepressants, and opioids.
- Increased sedation will occur with chamomile and valerian.

Implications for Physical Therapists

- Drugs will be extremely helpful in rehabilitation since they allow the therapist a more effective therapy.
- Patients starting drug therapy who have used extensor spasticity to maintain balance must be watched carefully while walking, because loss of this spasticity might compromise their balance and cause them to fall.
- Observe all patients carefully when they are walking or getting up, because drowsiness and muscle weakness can lead to falls.
- The physical therapist can best evaluate the effectiveness of treatment with these drugs and should share his or her evaluation with the physician to ensure that the best drug and dosage are used to the fullest benefit of the patient.
- Dichlorodifluoromethane spray should be applied from the muscle origin to insertion while the muscle is passively stretched. Never overcool the area. After warming, the spray can be reapplied.

References

1. APTA: American Physical Therapy Association: Guide to physical therapist practice, *Phys Ther*, 2001, The Association.
2. Behrman RE: *Nelson textbook of pediatrics*, ed 17, Philadelphia, 2004, W.B. Saunders.
3. Black JM, Hawks JH, Keene AM: *Medical-surgical nursing: Clinical management for positive outcomes*, ed 7, Philadelphia, 2005, W.B. Saunders.
4. Boissonnault W: *Primary care for the physical therapist: Examination and triage*, Philadelphia, 2005, Saunders.
5. Callen J, Greer K, Hood H, et al: *Color atlas of dermatology*, Philadelphia, 1993, W.B. Saunders.
6. Cameron MH: *Physical rehabilitation: Evidence-based examination, evaluation, and intervention*, Philadelphia, 2007, Saunders.
7. Cameron MH: *Physical agents in rehabilitation—from research to practice*, ed 3, Philadelphia, 2009, Saunders.
8. Chabner DE: *The language of medicine*, ed 8, Philadelphia, 2007, Saunders.
9. Chernecky CC: *Laboratory tests and diagnostic procedures*, ed 5, Philadelphia, 2008, Saunders.
10. Christensen BL: *Foundations and adult health nursing*, ed 5, St. Louis, 2006, Mosby.
11. Cioppa-Mosca J: *Postsurgical rehabilitation guidelines for the orthopedic clinician*, St. Louis, 2006, Mosby.
12. Cleland JA: *Orthopaedic clinical examination: An evidence-based approach for physical therapists*, Carlstadt, NJ, 2005, Icon Learning Systems.
13. Cohen J, Powderly WG: *Infectious diseases*, ed 2, St. Louis, 2004, Mosby.
14. Cook AM: *Cook and Hussey's assistive technologies: Principles and practice*, ed 3, St. Louis, 2008, Mosby.
15. Cummings NH: *Perspectives in athletic training*, St. Louis, 2009, Mosby.
16. Cuppett M: *General medical conditions in the athlete*, St. Louis, 2005, Mosby.
17. Current Procedural Terminology (CPT®), Chicago, 2007, American Medical Association.
18. Donatelli RA: *Sports-specific rehabilitation*. Philadelphia, 2007, Churchill Livingstone.
19. Drake RL: *Gray's anatomy for students*, London, 2005, Churchill Livingstone.
20. Forbes CD, Jackson WF: *Color atlas and text of clinical medicine*, ed 3, London, 2003, Mosby.
21. Frownfelter D: *Cardiovascular and pulmonary physical therapy: Evidence and practice*, ed 4, St. Louis, 2006, Mosby.
22. Gillen G: *Stroke rehabilitation: A function-based approach*, ed 2, St. Louis, 2004, Mosby.
23. Goldman L: *Cecil textbook of medicine*, ed 23, Philadelphia, 2008, W.B. Saunders.
24. Goodman CC: *Differential diagnosis for physical therapists: Screening for referral*, ed 4, Philadelphia, 2007, Saunders.
25. Goodman CC: *Pathology implications for the physical therapist*, ed 3, Philadelphia, 2009, Saunders.
26. Guyton AC: *Textbook of medical physiology*, ed 11, Philadelphia, 2006, Saunders.
27. Habif: *Clinical dermatology: A color guide to diagnosis and therapy*, ed 4, St. Louis, 2004, Mosby.

28. Hillegass E: *Essentials of cardiopulmonary physical therapy*, ed 2, Philadelphia, 2001, Saunders.
29. Hislop H, Montgomery J: *Daniels and Worthingham's muscle testing: Techniques of manual examination*, ed 8, Philadelphia, 2007, W.B. Saunders.
30. Hockenberry MJ: *Wong's essentials of pediatric nursing*, ed 8, St. Louis, 2009, Mosby.
31. Huber FE: *Therapeutic exercise: Treatment planning for progression*, ed 2, Philadelphia, 2006, Saunders.
32. Hurwitz S: *Clinical pediatric dermatology: A textbook of skin disorders of childhood and adolescence*, ed 2, Philadelphia, 1993, W.B. Saunders.
33. Ignatavicius DD, Workman ML: *Medical-surgical nursing: Critical thinking for collaborative care*, ed 5, Philadelphia, 2006, W.B. Saunders.
34. Jenkins DB: *Hollinshead's functional anatomy of the limbs and back*, ed 9. Philadelphia, 2009, Saunders.
35. Kliegman RM, Behrman RE: *Nelson textbook of pediatrics*, ed 18, Philadelphia, 2007, W.B. Saunders.
36. Kronenberg HM: *Williams textbook of endocrinology*, ed 11, Philadelphia, 2008, W.B. Saunders.
37. Lundy-Ekman L: *Neuroscience: Fundamentals for rehabilitation*, ed 3, Philadelphia, 2007, Saunders.
38. Lusardi MM: *Orthotics and prosthetics in rehabilitation*, ed 2, Philadelphia, 2006, W.B. Saunders.
39. Magee DJ: *Orthopedic physical assessment*, ed 5, Philadelphia, 2008, Saunders.
40. Mandell GL: *Principles and practice of infectious disease*, ed 6, London, 2005, Churchill Livingstone.
41. Manske RC: *Postsurgical orthopedic sports rehabilitation: Knee & shoulder*, St. Louis, 2006, Mosby.
42. Martin S: *Neurologic interventions for physical therapy*, ed 2, Philadelphia, 2007, Saunders.
43. Marx JM, Hockberger R: *Rosen's emergency medicine: Concepts and clinical practice*, ed 6, St. Louis, 2006, Mosby.
44. Maxey L, Magnusson J: *Rehabilitation of the post surgical orthopedic patient*, St. Louis, 2007, Mosby.
45. *Mosby's medical, nursing, and allied health dictionary*, ed 6, St. Louis, 2002, Mosby.
46. National Heart Lung and Blood Institute (www.nhlbi.nih.gov/), Bethesda, MD.
47. National Institutes of Health (www.nih.gov/), Bethesda, MD.
48. Neumann DA: *Kinesiology of the musculoskeletal system: Foundations for physical rehabilitation*, ed 2, St. Louis, 2010, Mosby.
49. NIH Clinical Center (clinicalcenter.nih.gov/), Bethesda, MD.
50. Noble J: Textbook of primary care medicine, ed 3. St. Louis, 2001, Mosby.
51. O'Shea RK: *Pediatrics for the physical therapist assistant*, Philadelphia, 2009, Saunders.
52. Olson DA: *Clinician's guide to assistive technology*, St. Louis, 2001, Mosby.
53. Olson KA: *Manual physical therapy of the spine*, Philadelphia, 2009, Saunders.
54. Pagliarulo M: *Introduction to physical therapy*, ed 3, St. Louis, 2007, Mosby.
55. Pendleton HM: *Pedretti's occupational therapy: Practice skills for physical dysfunction*, ed 6, St. Louis, 2006, Mosby.
56. Pierson FM: *Principles & techniques of patient care*, ed 4, Philadelphia, 2008, Saunders.
57. Placzek JD: *Orthopaedic physical therapy secrets*, ed 2, St. Louis, 2006, Mosby.
58. Rakel: *Textbook of family medicine*, ed 7, Philadelphia, 2007, Saunders.
59. Reese NB: *Muscle and sensory testing*, ed 2, Philadelphia, 2005, Saunders.
60. Reese NB, Bandy W: *Joint range of motion and muscle length testing*, Philadelphia, 2002, Saunders.

61. Seidel HM: *Mosby's guide to physical examination*, ed 6, St. Louis, 2006, Mosby.
62. Sisto SA: *Spinal cord injuries: Management and rehabilitation*, St. Louis, 2009, Mosby.
63. Swartz M: *Textbook of physical diagnosis: History and examination*, ed 5, Philadelphia, 2006, Saunders.
64. Tan JC: *Practice manual of physical medicine and rehabilitation*, ed 2, St. Louis, 2006, Mosby.
65. Thibodeau GA: *Anatomy & physiology*, ed 6, St. Louis, 2007, Mosby.
66. Umphred DA: *Neurological rehabilitation*, ed 5, St. Louis, 2006, Mosby.
67. Watchie J: *Cardiopulmonary physical therapy*, ed 2, Philadelphia, Saunders, in press.
68. Zitelli BJ, Davis HW: *Atlas of pediatric physical diagnosis*, St. Louis, 2002, Mosby.

Index

Page numbers followed by f indicate figures; t, tables.